The Mayo Clinic Diet

SECOND EDITION

Mayo Clinic

MEDICAL EDITOR
Donald D. Hensrud, M.D., M.P.H.

EDITORIAL DIRECTOR
Paula M. Marlow Limbeck

SENIOR EDITOR
Karen R. Wallevand

PRODUCT MANAGER
Christopher C. Frye

ART DIRECTOR
Stewart Jay Koski

ILLUSTRATION, PHOTOGRAPHY AND PRODUCTION
Kent McDaniel, Matthew C. Meyer, Gunnar T. Soroos, Malgorzata (Gosha) B. Weivoda

PROOFREADING
Miranda M. Attlesey, Alison K. Baker, Julie M. Maas

INDEXING
Steve Rath

CONTRIBUTORS
Rachel A. Haring Bartony, Matthew M. Clark, Ph.D., L.P., Lisa M. Dierks, RDN, Ryan J. Eastman, Jason S. Ewoldt, RDN, Philip T. Hagen, M.D., Jessica R. Holst, RDN, Michael D. Jensen, M.D., Sara M. Link, Angela L. Murad, RDN, Deborah J. Rhodes, M.D., Kristine R. Schmitz, RDN, Warren G. Thompson, M.D., Kristen S. Vickers Douglas, Ph.D., L.P., Laura Hamilton Waxman, Jennifer A. Welper

Each of the habits in *Lose It!* has been the subject of scientific studies that support its role in weight management. In addition, Mayo Clinic conducted a two-week program to test the validity of this habit-based approach to quick weight loss. The 33 women who completed the program lost an average of 6.59 pounds, with individual results varying from 0.2 to 13.8 pounds lost. The 14 men who completed the program lost an average of 9.97 pounds, with individual results varying from 5.2 to 18.8 pounds lost. Individual results will vary. Consult your doctor before starting any diet program.

Published by Mayo Clinic

For bulk sales to employers, member groups and health-related companies, write Mayo Clinic, 200 First St. SW, Rochester, MN 55905, call 800-430-9699, or email *SpecialSalesMayoBooks@mayo.edu*.

ISBN 978-1-945564-00-0

Library of Congress Control Number: 2016946652

Second Edition

Printed in the USA

1 2 3 4 5 6 7 8 9 10

Jacket design by Paul E. Krause

Table of contents

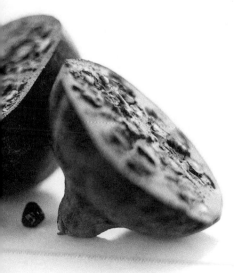

Table of contents (continued)

Part 1 *Lose It!*

All you have to do to lose weight during this two-week period is:

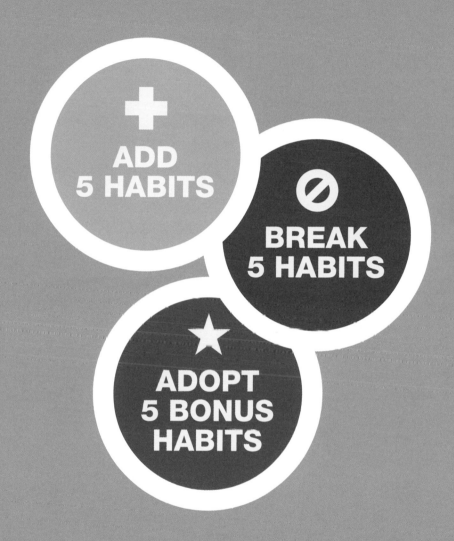

ADD 5 HABITS

BREAK 5 HABITS

ADOPT 5 BONUS HABITS

It's that simple. Get Started!

What is The Mayo Clinic Diet?

People often say they're 'on a diet' to lose weight. This often implies something that's rigid, focuses on what you can't eat, and that's a negative experience. Therefore, it's not surprising, that most people eventually go 'off' their diets and soon regain any weight they may have lost.

The Mayo Clinic Diet is a different type of weight-loss program. It's not an 'on again, off again' diet. It's a lifestyle approach designed to help you lose weight, improve your health, and feel better. The program is designed to be practical and enjoyable so that you'll with stick with it for the long haul.

The two main principles of *The Mayo Clinic Diet* are to follow an eating plan that's low in calories yet tasty and satisfying, and to burn more calories through physical activity.

You'll jump right in and start losing weight in the first phase of the diet — the *Lose It!* phase — which lasts two weeks. You'll continue your weight loss journey in the second phase of the diet — the *Live It!* phase — that will hopefully last the rest of your life.

It's important to us that you improve your health while losing weight. Not all diets will do that. For example, if you follow a very restrictive 800-calorie diet of primarily cabbage soup (yes, it's been tried!) you'll lose weight, but your health won't improve. And chances are, you won't enjoy it.

The Mayo Clinic Diet is structured to improve your health and reduce your risk of chronic diseases such as heart disease, cancer and diabetes. It's also designed to help you feel good — to have more energy and not feel fatigued all the time. We want to help you get back that spring in your step and that sparkle in your eye.

As you'll soon learn, this approach to weight loss is very practical and flexible. We provide you the knowledge and tools you need to make important lifestyle changes, but we don't tell you exactly what to do.

You know yourself best, so it's up to you to create your own personal weight-loss program. We give you many suggestions, but you're the one to decide what you'll do and when you'll do it.

Two Phases: *Lose It!* and *Live It!*

Most people wanting to lose weight want to lose it quickly. We get that. That's why we designed the first part of the diet — the first two weeks — as a jump-start period. During this time, you can lose 6 to 10 pounds by making some sudden changes in your habits.

We reviewed the medical literature, did some testing, and came up with 15 habits associated with safe and healthy weight loss. In fact, we believe the *Lose It!* phase is the healthiest way to quickly lose weight there is.

Initially, these habit changes may seem daunting. But as the weight starts to come off, people become empowered and realize that they can actually do it (remember, it's only two weeks!).

The *Live It!* phase of *The Mayo Clinic Diet* is a continuation of *Lose It!*, but it's intended for the long haul. Here, you create a personal lifestyle program to help you lose about 1 to 2 pounds a week. The changes you make also will help you to maintain your weight once you reach your weight-loss goal.

Live It! provides more overall structure, but we try to keeps things flexible so that you can adapt the program to your own 'tastes.'

What people really like is that you don't need to count calories, and you don't need to measure — no food scales or calculators are needed! Instead, we teach you easy ways to estimate servings and how much food from each of the food groups you should eat each day.

We understand that change can be challenging, but losing weight doesn't have to be difficult or boring. Many people find the longer they follow the program tho easier and more rewarding it becomes. New lifestyle habits replace old ones to create a healthier and happier you!

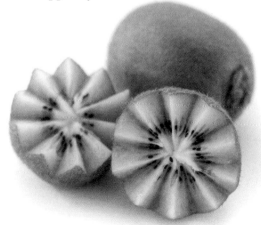

Chapter 1
Ready, set, go

You want to lose weight, so let's get going. *Lose It!* is designed to help you safely lose 6 to 10 pounds in two weeks and jump-start your journey to a healthier you. How much you lose is ultimately your call — the more closely you follow *Lose It!*, the more you'll likely lose. This chapter provides some necessary preliminaries before you dive in.

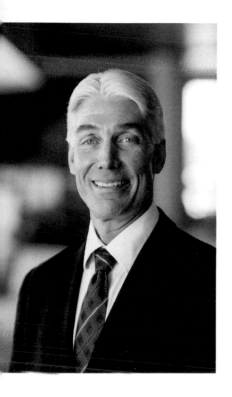

**Donald D. Hensrud,
M.D., M.P.H.**

Preventive Medicine

How are you feeling? Hopeful? Cautiously optimistic? Wondering if this is the program that will finally help you get healthy?

As you know, losing weight and keeping it off isn't easy. If it were, people wouldn't be struggling as much as they are — more than two-thirds of adults in the United States are overweight or obese.

Because weight is such a challenging issue that affects so many people, there are many programs out there that promise quick, effortless weight loss. Sometimes they work for a short while, but, really, how much cabbage soup can you eat?!

The Mayo Clinic Diet requires some planning and effort, and it involves opening yourself up to new ways of eating and being active — lifestyle changes. But these changes aren't drudgery. And most importantly, for the time and effort you invest, the potential rewards you'll experience to your health and quality of life are tremendous.

Our goal is to help you achieve both a healthier weight and a healthier lifestyle. This is not only possible, but very achievable. By embracing these lifestyle changes your health risks will decrease, your weight will improve, and you'll feel much better — about your weight and about yourself.

We will be your partner in this journey. Good luck, and let's hit the road!

Are you ready?

Time now to get down to business. You're eager to get started and so are we! You can read more about the philosophy of the diet and why and how it works in later chapters.

First up, are you ready? There's a good time to start losing weight, and there's a bad time. You don't want to put off your start date any longer than necessary, but you also don't want to set yourself up for failure by trying to diet at a time when you're facing a lot of obstacles.

On pages 14 and 15 is a short quiz to determine if now is a good time to make big changes to your daily routine. Turn to the quiz and answer the questions honestly.

If your results indicate that this isn't a good time to try to lose weight, address those factors interfering with your plans. Try to deal with them promptly so that you can start soon.

If now is a good time to begin (and we hope it is!), keep reading.

Before you start

Before you begin your diet, you want to make sure that you're prepared. The more prepared you are, the better your chances of success. Take these steps:

+ **Know the plan.** Read Chapters 1-5 so you know what's ahead.

+ **Pick a start date.** Don't make the date too far away or you might lose your motivation. On your start date, jump in and begin!

+ **Ready your kitchen.** Get rid of all of the food you don't want to eat and stock your pantry and refrigerator with more-healthy options, such as plenty of fruits and vegetables.

+ **Line up your gear.** Make sure you have a good pair of walking shoes, comfortable clothes and whatever else you need to be physically active.

+ **Set up a tracking system.** You'll need a way to track how well you did following the habits. You can photocopy the habit tracker on page 19. You can use *The Mayo Clinic*

Diet Journal that accompanies this book. Or you can develop your own system. You'll also need a way to log your daily and weekly goals. **JOT IT** ▸

+ **Get mentally prepared.** Just like athletes do before a big game, get yourself psyched to begin. Tell yourself that you can do this (because you can!), and think of all of the positive things that will come from this new venture.

Finding your inner motivation

Odds are, you already have a pretty good idea of what you need to do to lose weight — eat less and move more. But if you're reading this book, you probably haven't done it. Why?

Likely because you haven't found the necessary motivation.

Knowing the how-to-do-it, what-to-eat, and what-not-to-eat concepts of weight loss are certainly important. But the most critical element of weight loss is what *you* bring to the table — your own personal drive to succeed.

Use *The Mayo Clinic Diet Journal*, a notebook, a cellphone app, an online tool or whatever works best for you to track how well you followed key habits to healthy weight loss and record your progress.

The *Jot It* icon above is used throughout the book to remind you to record your food servings and activities.

In Chapter 11, you can read why food and activity records, as well as tracking your weight, will help you in the long run.

Apps and online tools that allow you to log your food intake and daily activities are constantly changing. Use whatever tracking system works for you.

Readiness quiz

Circle one best answer for each question.

❶ How motivated are you to lose weight?

a. Highly motivated

b. Moderately motivated

c. Somewhat motivated

d. Slightly motivated or not at all

❷ Considering the amount of stress affecting your life right now, to what extent can you focus on weight loss and on making lifestyle changes?

a. Can focus easily

b. Can focus relatively well

c. Uncertain

d. Can focus somewhat or not at all

❸ Initially, people often lose weight quickly. But over the long run, it's best to lose weight at a rate of 1 to 2 pounds a week. How realistic are your expectations about how much weight you'd like to lose and how fast you want to lose it?

a. Very realistic

b. Moderately realistic

c. Somewhat realistic

d. Somewhat or very unrealistic

❹ Aside from special celebrations, do you ever eat a lot of food rapidly while feeling that your eating is out of control?

a. No

d. Yes

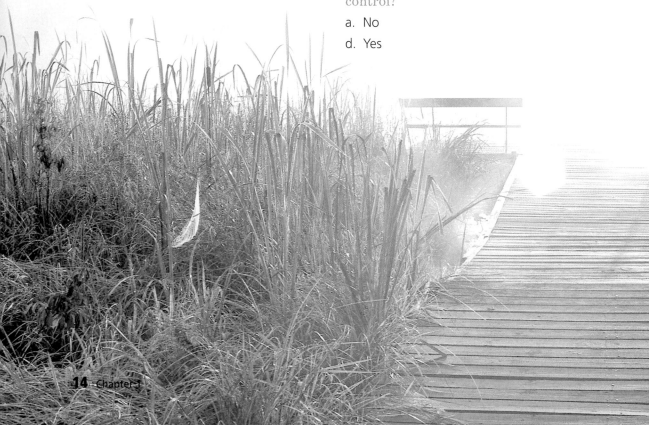

❺ If you answered yes to the previous question, how often have you eaten like this during the last year?

a. About once a month or less
b. A few times a month
c. About once a week
d. About three times a week or more

❻ Do you eat for emotional reasons, for example, when you feel anxious, depressed, angry or lonely?

a. Never or rarely
b. Occasionally
c. Frequently
d. Always

❼ How confident are you that you can make changes in your eating habits and maintain them?

a Completely confident
b. Moderately confident
c. Somewhat confident
d. Slightly or not at all confident

❽ How confident are you that you can exercise several times a week?

a. Completely confident
b. Moderately confident
c. Somewhat confident
d. Slightly or not at all confident

If most of your responses are:

+ **a and b,** then you're probably ready to start a weight-loss program.
+ **b and c,** consider whether you're ready or if you should wait and take action to prepare yourself.
+ **d,** you may want to hold off on your start date and take steps to prepare yourself. Re-assess your readiness again soon. You may want to talk to your doctor about what you can do to increase your readiness.

Note: If your answer to question 5 was b, c or d, discuss this with your doctor. If you have an eating disorder, it's crucial that you get appropriate treatment.

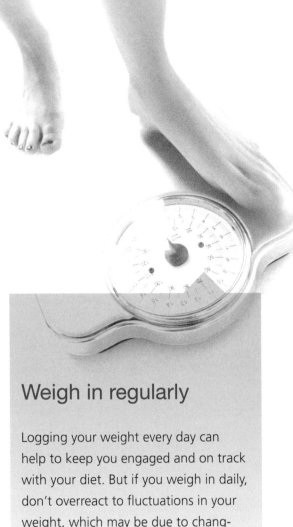

To be successful at losing weight, you need to figure out what your motivation is — what will give you an *ongoing, burning desire* to keep at it.

Start by asking yourself this: "Why do I want to lose weight?" There may be several reasons. Improved health. More energy. Better beach bod. Make a list of what's *important to you*.

For example, let's say your top reason for losing weight is that you have a high school reunion coming up and you don't want to be embarrassed (OK, maybe that's not as important as improving your health, but let's run with it). Under that you write, "Show Bobby Jones (the boy who dumped you) what he missed," or "Not feel like a blimp on the dance floor." There are no wrong answers here. What matters to you is what's most important.

Keep these motivators in front of you — especially at moments of decision ("Do I eat that sweet roll or not?"). Maybe you use notes posted around your home and office, reminders on your cellphone or a photo of yourself as you want (or don't want) to look.

Weigh in regularly

Logging your weight every day can help to keep you engaged and on track with your diet. But if you weigh in daily, don't overreact to fluctuations in your weight, which may be due to changing body fluid levels rather than gains or losses in body fat. Weigh yourself at least once a week, and look for trends over several days or weeks.

Be creative. Just as you came up with your own motivators, use your own problem-solving skills to find ways to keep your motivation fresh.

Your starting point

Before you begin *The Mayo Clinic Diet*, identify your starting point: **JOT IT** ▸

+ **Record your initial weight.** Weigh yourself at a time and in a manner you'll be able to follow consistently, such as right after getting up in the morning.

+ **Determine your body mass index.** BMI is a better indicator of body fat than is body weight. See the table on page 145 to determine your BMI. Write it down for future comparison.

+ **Measure your waist.** Use a flexible tape and measure around your waist just above the highest points on your hipbones. Record the result.

You'll also want to:

+ **Consider your health.** If you have health issues, such as diabetes, heart disease, shortness of breath or joint disease, are pregnant, or have any questions about your health, see your doctor before beginning this or any weight management program.

Talk to your doctor

Big changes in diet and exercise and rapid weight loss can sometimes lead to symptoms such as dizziness and fatigue or can necessitate changes in medications. If you experience these symptoms while on *The Mayo Clinic Diet* or are taking medications, talk to your doctor.

Some final thoughts

Once you've completed these steps, you're ready to roll.

A few final words about *Lose It!*. Sometimes people make these two weeks more difficult than they need to be. Remember, you don't need to count calories and you don't need to adhere to a bunch of rigid rules.

Just do what the habits recommend. For example, eat a healthy breakfast. Don't worry about *exactly* what or how much, as long as you follow the habits.

Chances are, certain behaviors got you to this point — eating fast food for lunch, having ice cream before bed, not exercising. Most people don't realize how much certain behaviors, taken together, help pack on pounds. Bad habits are easy to get into and hard to break — but not impossible!

If you do what's recommended these next two weeks, you'll be avoiding many of the things that likely led to your weight gain. In other words, you'll be abandoning many of your unhealthy habits. And that's how you're going to lose weight.

The focus of this diet is on changing your habits — getting rid of the unhealthy behaviors that ultimately led to your weight gain and replacing them with healthy new ones.

Over these next two weeks, realize that no one is perfect. Few people can follow all 15 habits the full two weeks. But give it your best shot. You may be surprised by how many of the habits you can achieve, and you may find the changes really aren't as difficult as you anticipated.

On your start date, begin!

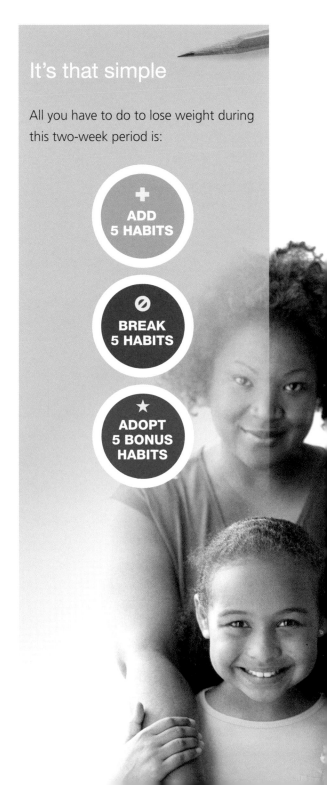

It's that simple

All you have to do to lose weight during this two-week period is:

+ ADD 5 HABITS

⊘ BREAK 5 HABITS

★ ADOPT 5 BONUS HABITS

Habit tracker

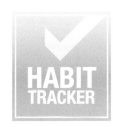

✔ **Check if done**

	Day 1	Day 2	Day 3	Day 4	Day 5	Day 6	Day 7	TOTALS
ADD 5 HABITS								
1. Eat a healthy breakfast								
2. Eat vegetables and fruits								
3. Eat whole grains								
4. Eat healthy fats								
5. Move!								
BREAK 5 HABITS								
1. No TV while eating								
2. No sugar								
3. No snacks								
4. Only moderate meat and dairy								
5. No eating at restaurants								
5 BONUS HABITS								
1. Keep diet records								
2. Keep exercise/activity records								
3. Move more!								
4. Eat "real" food								
5. Write your daily goals								
TOTALS:								

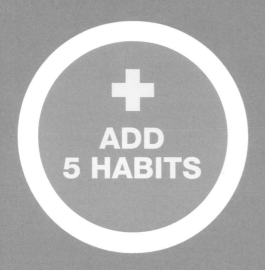

ADD
5 HABITS

Chapter 2
Add 5 Habits

Changing habits can be challenging, and people often underestimate how difficult it can be to alter their everyday patterns. But what's often challenging to begin with generally becomes more manageable over time. In other words, stick with it, because it will get better. In this chapter, we discuss five habits to build into your daily routine to kick-start your weight-loss plan.

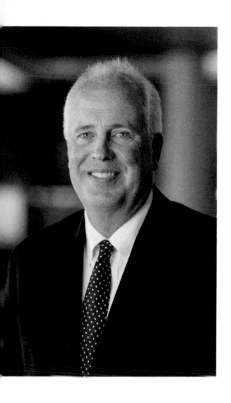

**Matthew M. Clark,
Ph.D., L.P.**
Psychology

So often when people are trying to lose weight, their focus is on what they can't do or what they need to give up. For example: "I can't have fast food for lunch anymore." "There goes eating chocolate when I'm stressed." "I'll miss my buttered popcorn on movie night."

These are positive lifestyle changes, but the attention is being given to what these individuals are giving up — not what they're gaining. It's not uncommon for people to share with me the real loss they feel.

This chapter isn't about what you need to give up, but what you want to add to your day. You're given strategies for how to incorporate five healthy behaviors into your daily routine. Keep in mind that new behaviors take time. These changes may not come automatically or be easy, but I encourage you to give them your best effort. And by concentrating on what you're adding, you'll pay less attention to what you're giving up.

Succeeding long term with weight loss isn't just about eliminating negative behaviors but changing how you go about your day to avoid difficult situations. If you're a stress eater, yes, you want to stop reaching for a candy bar whenever you feel stressed, but by building exercise into your daily routine, you can lower your stress level so that you're less likely to be placed in this type of high-stress situation.

Do your best to embrace these changes — remember, no matter how big or small, positive changes add up.

ADD 1

Eat a healthy breakfast

but not too much

What:
Have breakfast every morning. You don't need to eat a lot — just something to get you off to a good start.

Why:
Research shows that people who eat a healthy breakfast manage their weight better than do people who don't eat breakfast. Breakfast is associated with improved performance at school and work, and it helps prevent you from becoming ravenous later in the day.

+ Keep it whole. Try whole grains, such as oatmeal, whole-grain cold cereal, whole-grain toast.

+ Include some color. Add some fresh or frozen unsweetened fruit.

+ Make it filling. Low-fat milk and yogurt, an egg, nuts, seeds, and nut butters such as peanut butter can help you feel satisfied throughout the morning.

+ Plan ahead. If time is an issue, place a box of cereal, a bowl and a spoon on the table the evening before.

+ Choose wisely. Select your cereal — hot or cold — by checking the Nutrition Facts label for fiber (choose more) and sugar (choose less). If you add milk or yogurt, choose reduced-fat or fat-free varieties. Top with banana slices or berries.

+ Mix it up. Try a smoothie made with fruit (bananas, pineapple, fresh or frozen berries) and low-fat yogurt. Blend the ingredients to a smooth consistency.

+ Bring it with. Keep handy items that you can grab and take with you to work. Convenient foods include apples, oranges, bananas, pre-portioned cereals, low-fat yogurt in single-serving containers, whole-grain bagels (mini-sized) and low-fat cottage cheese in single-serving containers. Stir in berries or fruit to add fiber and sweetness.

+ Wrap it up. Make a breakfast wrap with whole-wheat tortillas, roll in scrambled eggs with diced peppers and onions, or peanut butter and bananas.

+ Make it healthy. For French toast, use whole-grain bread, egg whites or an egg substitute, a pinch of cinnamon, and a few drops of vanilla extract for sweetness. Fry on a nonstick skillet or use a cooking spray. Top with unsweetened applesauce, berries or sliced bananas.

+ Innovate. If you don't like traditional breakfast foods, eat something healthy that you do like. For example, fix yourself a sandwich made with lean meat, low-fat cheese, vegetables and whole-grain bread.

If you're not in the habit of eating breakfast, start out small. Grab a piece of fruit or a healthy granola bar. Gradually include other food groups. Just like you got used to not eating breakfast, you can get used to eating breakfast. With time, you'll begin to feel hungry in the morning.

When you don't eat breakfast, your body says, "If you're not going to feed me, I won't be hungry," and you don't miss eating in the morning. However, you tend to make up for this by overeating later in the day. Eating breakfast helps you lose weight by reducing the urge to overeat later in the day.

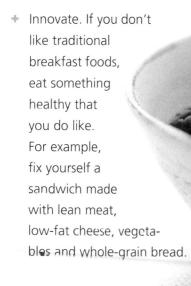

ADD 2

Eat vegetables and fruits

4 or more servings of vegetables and 3 or more of fruits

What:
Eat at least four servings of vegetables and three servings of fruits every day. What's a serving? See pages 256-283.

Why:
Fresh vegetables and fruits are the foundation of a healthy diet and successful weight loss. Most processed foods, sweets and nondiet sodas contain a lot of calories in just a small portion. Vegetables and fruits are the opposite — they have lots of bulk and few calories. You can eat a lot, consume fewer calories and feel full at the end of your meal.

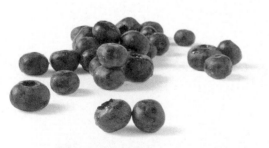

+ Be selective. Eat only those vegetables and fruits that you like, but don't be afraid to explore different types and varieties. You may be surprised by their appealing tastes and textures.

+ Make them No. 1. Vegetables should take up the largest portion of your dinner plate, with fruits trailing close behind. Eat these foods first, rather than reserving them for the end of the meal.

+ Consider them a priority. When planning meals, think of dishes that contain vegetables or fruits as the centerpiece and build the rest of your meal around them.

+ Mix it up. Try both raw and cooked vegetables. Lightly cook, steam or roast vegetables for a softer texture. Sprinkle them with herbs for flavor.

+ Use 'em as grab-and-go foods. When you're in a hurry, have ready-to-eat vegetables and fruits on hand. Buy fresh vegetables and fruits that require little preparation, such as baby carrots, cherry tomatoes, bananas and grapes.

+ Think toppings. Add bananas, strawberries or other fruit to cereal or yogurt.

- Go for fresh. Dried fruit and fruit juice are higher in calories than fresh or un-sweetened frozen fruit, so the "unlimited servings" rule doesn't apply to them. Dried fruits and fruits juices can significantly increase your calorie intake.

- Explore. Visit local farmers markets. The freshness and variety may encourage you to try new kinds of produce. Farmers markets also are a great place to build a sense of community.

- Innovate. Find ways to incorporate vegetables with other foods or into existing recipes. Add them to soups, casseroles and pizzas, and pile them onto sandwiches.

- Pack 'em. When traveling, snack on ready-to-eat vegetables and fruits.

YES, I CAN!

On this program, you'll find that the more veggies and fruits you eat, the fewer high-calorie foods you'll consume. That's why it's OK to eat as many vegetables and fruits as you want. Make sure to have them available to you at all times, and when you're hungry, eat some.

ADD 3

Eat whole grains

such as whole-grain bread, oatmeal and brown rice

What:
Eat whole-grain breads and pastas, brown rice, oatmeal, and other whole-grain products, instead of white, refined and highly processed foods.

Why:
Whole grains include the entire grain kernel, which is packed with essential vitamins, minerals and fiber that are part of a healthy diet. Whole grains help you feel full by adding fiber and bulk, and they help reduce your risk of becoming overweight.

+ Start whole. For breakfast, have whole-grain cereal, such as oatmeal or a bran cereal, or eat whole-grain toast instead of white.

+ Stock up. Fill your pantry with whole-grain products. This includes whole-grain brown and wild rice, whole-grain pastas, and whole-grain cereals that aren't sweetened (if you want sweetness, pile on fruit). Also include on your list oatmeal, pita bread and whole-grain bagels.

+ Go brown. Use brown rice as a healthy alternative to white rice. If you want it fast, buy instant brown rice.

+ Think main meal. Prepare a meatless main dish made from whole grains, such as whole-wheat spinach lasagna, red beans over brown rice, whole-wheat spaghetti with marinara sauce, or vegetable stir-fry over brown rice.

+ Experiment. Include side dishes that use products such as bulgur, kasha or whole-grain barley.

+ Throw 'em in. Add whole-grain barley or wild rice to soups, stews and casseroles.

- Do a flour swap. Substitute whole-grain flour for half the white flour in recipes for pancakes, waffles, muffins and bread.

- Look at the label. When shopping, look at the food label for specific terms such as *whole wheat*, *whole oats* or *brown rice*. Terms such as *100% wheat*, *multigrain* and *stone-ground* do not mean the product contains whole grains.

Worried about gluten?

Gluten is a protein mixture found in wheat, barley and rye. It's what gives structure to pasta, bread and other baked goods, and it's found in a lot of things you eat.

Some people have trouble digesting gluten. Celiac disease and non-celiac gluten sensitivity are two gluten-related conditions that have received a lot of attention. If you're among those who can't eat gluten, know that not all grains contain gluten. Look for products labeled gluten-free or products made from grains naturally free of gluten, such as buckwheat, cornmeal, flax, quinoa, and brown and wild rice.

If you can eat gluten, do so! Don't avoid gluten because of the increase in gluten-free foods. Whole grains that contain gluten are associated with many health benefits.

ADD 4

Eat healthy fats

such as olive oil, vegetable oils and nuts

What:
When consuming fat, make healthy choices — olive oil, vegetable oils, avocados, nuts and nut butters, and the oils that come from nuts.

Why:
These fats are the most heart healthy. But don't forget that all fats contain about the same number of calories, so even healthier fats need to be consumed sparingly as part of a healthy diet.

+ Check food labels. Compare similar foods and choose the one that's lower in fat. Make sure it's also lower in calories — some low-fat and fat-free foods are higher in sugar and not much lower in calories. Some also are high in sodium.

+ Choose wisely. The types of fat in commercially made products are listed on Nutrition Facts labels. Limit foods high in saturated fat and trans fat, and select foods made with unsaturated fats (polyunsaturated and monounsaturated).

+ Limit dairy products. To reduce saturated fat, choose reduced-fat or fat-free milk, yogurt, sour cream, cheese, and other dairy products.

+ Avoid trans fats. They're the most unhealthy. Manufacturers are limiting their use, but check labels as a precaution. Trans fats are most common in stick margarine and vegetable shortening and processed products made from them.

+ Forgo frying. Use low-fat cooking techniques such as grilling, broiling, baking, roasting or steaming. A good-quality nonstick pan may allow you to cook food without using oil or butter. You can also try cooking spray, low-sodium broth or water instead of using cooking oil.

+ Cut out the fat. Choose meat with the least amount of visible fat, and trim most of the fat from the edges of the meat. Remove all skin from poultry before cooking it or buy skinless breasts. Even small amounts of lean meat and poultry contain fat.

Fats: They're not all the same

Monounsaturated and polyunsaturated fats are the best choices. Look for products with little or no saturated fats, and avoid trans fats. Saturated and trans fats increase blood cholesterol levels. Remember that all fats are high in calories.

+ *Monounsaturated fats* are found in olive, canola and peanut oils, as well as most nuts and avocados.
+ *Polyunsaturated fats* are found in other plant-based oils, such as safflower, corn, sunflower, soybean, sesame and cottonseed oils.
+ *Saturated fats* are found in animal-based foods, such as meats, poultry, lard, egg yolks and whole-fat dairy products (including butter and cheese). They're also in cocoa butter and coconut, palm and other tropical oils, which are used in many coffee lighteners, snack crackers, baked goods and other processed foods.
+ *Trans fats* — also called hydrogenated vegetable oil — may be found in hardened vegetable fats, such as stick margarine and vegetable shortening, and in foods made with them (including many crackers, cookies, cakes, pies and other baked goods, as well as many candies, snack foods and french fries).

+ ADD 5

Move!

walk or exercise for 30 minutes or more every day

 What:
Every day, include at least 30 minutes of physical activity or exercise in your schedule.

Why:
Physical activity burns calories, and too much sitting isn't good for you. The more physically active you are, the more calories you burn. Physical activity, including exercise, has a great number of health benefits.

HOW

+ Choose what you like. The best exercise is the one you'll do consistently.

+ Be flexible. The best time to exercise is whenever you can.

+ All movement counts. Walking to the store, weeding the garden and cleaning the house count as physical activity.

+ Break it up. Three 10-minute sessions of brisk walking can provide almost the same benefits that one 30-minute session does.

+ Plan activity breaks. Include time in your day to stretch and move around. Walk to get some water. Walk up and down a few flights of stairs.

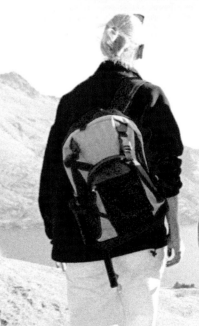

- Don't overdo it. If you've been inactive, start slowly and give your body a chance to get used to increased activity. A common mistake is starting an activity program at too high an intensity.

- Find ways to move. When you talk on the phone or check your email, stand instead of sit. When watching your favorite TV program or reading a book, walk on a treadmill or pedal a stationary bike.

- Mix it up. Try new types of exercise and don't feel tied to one activity.

- Find a partner. Having a partner will make exercise more fun, and it will help you stick with your activity plan.

The hardest part about physical activity often is getting started — putting on your shoes and getting out the door to walk or run. Psych yourself up with positive self-talk to overcome any hesitation when you're deciding whether or not to exercise.

Positive self-talk tips

- Instead of, "I'm so tired," tell yourself, "I'll feel so energized when I'm done."
- Instead of, "I should be better at this by now," tell yourself, "I'm making steady progress."
- Instead of, "Skipping this one won't matter," tell yourself, "Every little bit makes a difference."
- Instead of, "I'll never stick with this exercise program," tell yourself, "Take one day at a time."

From the Mayo Clinic Healthy Weight Pyramid ...

Throughout *The Mayo Clinic Diet*, use the Mayo Clinic Healthy Weight Pyramid as your guide to making smart eating choices. There's detailed information on the pyramid in Chapters 9 and 15, but what you need to start doing now is eat more foods from the food groups at the base of the pyramid and less from those at the top — and start moving more. At this point, don't worry about being too precise. In later chapters, we'll get into more specifics on how to use the pyramid to help plan your daily meals.

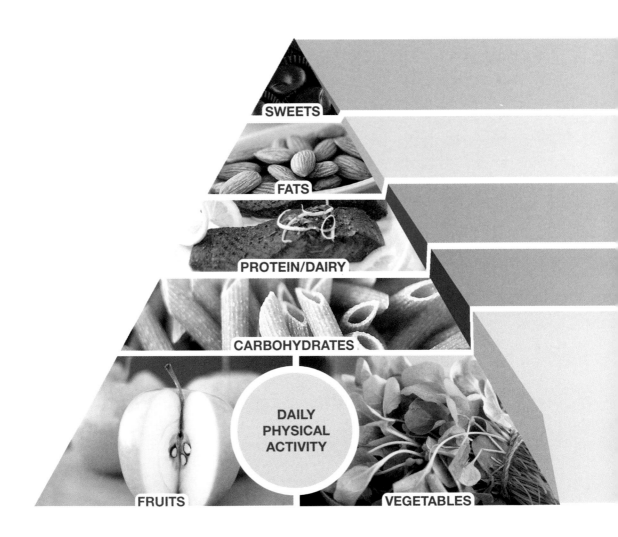

SWEETS

FATS

PROTEIN/DAIRY

CARBOHYDRATES

DAILY PHYSICAL ACTIVITY

FRUITS

VEGETABLES

to the Mayo Clinic Healthy Dining Table

Below is how a meal might look when you follow the pyramid. Vegetables and fruits should make up the largest portion of your meal. An easy way to include more vegetables in your diet is to have a green salad with your meal. Other foods should be eaten in moderation. Limit carbohydrates to a quarter of your plate. The same for protein and dairy. Fats and sweets should be eaten sparingly and they may not be a part of every meal. For your fluids, include beverages that are low in calories or calorie-free.

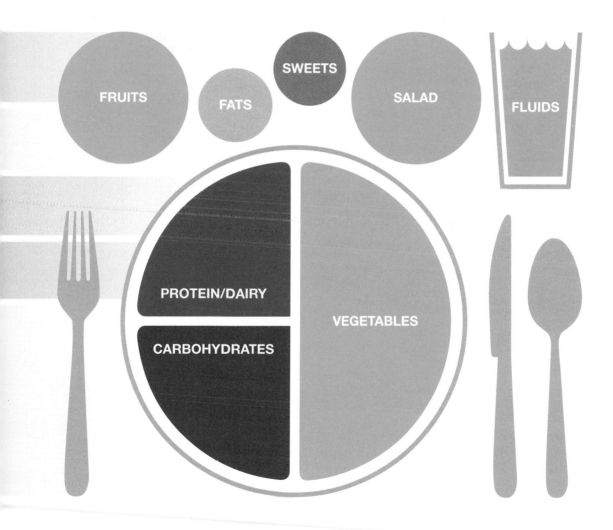

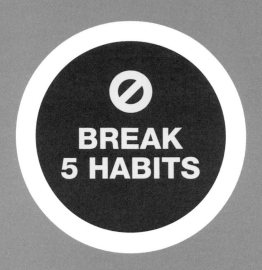

**BREAK
5 HABITS**

Chapter 3
Break 5 Habits

Changing any habit can be challenging, but reprogramming yourself to stop doing something that you've been doing for many years — that affects you emotionally, socially and psychologically — can be especially difficult. Here are five habits to break that may be a little tough to swallow, but that can make a big difference in your weight.

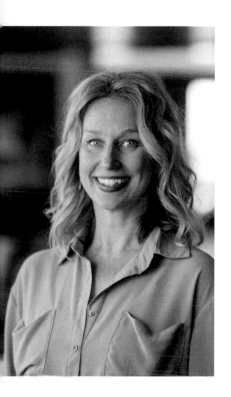

Kristen S. Vickers Douglas, Ph.D., L.P.
Psychology

OK, brace yourself. This part is challenging. But this is where you really learn about how and why you eat. Think of these changes as small experiments that provide an opportunity to learn about you.

Like many people, you likely use food as a pick-me-up — for energy, to boost your mood, for fun, for something to do when you're bored. Eating is social and emotional and it impacts our mind and body, for better and worse. Don't get frustrated if you think these changes are too hard. Focus instead on what you're feeling and learning. Perhaps you feel cranky and deprived the first few days you don't have sugar ... but then what? Do you and your body learn to adjust?

For two weeks, go for it and take advantage of this opportunity. Then, with the new data you collect, figure out which of these habits you want to continue to work on. Adopting new habits can be tough. Sometimes, though, tolerating a little discomfort is what we need. No, we don't want you to be miserable, starving and cranky. But allowing yourself to feel frustrated, bored or sad, and not turn to food to satisfy those emotions, can help you become stronger.

Be kind to yourself, but push yourself a bit. You'll never know what you're truly capable of unless you try. And remember you don't have to be perfect. If you mess this up, well, then welcome to the club of imperfect human beings. Gather up your strength and keep going!

BREAK 1

No TV while eating

and only as much TV time as time you spend exercising

What:
Don't watch TV while eating (or, flipping it around, no eating while watching TV). The same applies for any "screen time," such as cellphone and computer use. And spend only as much time watching TV as you do exercising.

Why:
Studies show that too much screen time contributes to increased health risks and increased weight — you aren't moving, and there's also a good chance that you're sipping or nibbling on something. If you establish the rule of no TV or screen time while eating, and only as much time watching TV as time you spend exercising, you're breaking one bad habit (mindless nibbling) while developing a good one (being more active).

+ Use sticky notes. Put a sticky on the TV and the remote control to remind yourself that you need to exercise before watching TV or while watching TV.

+ Don't forget other devices. The same rule applies to other devices such as your computer and iPad.

+ Earn your time. Build up TV and screen time by exercising beforehand. Don't use TV minutes before you've earned them.

+ Eat without distraction. No TV, computer or cellphone while eating. You're more likely to overeat if you get lost in what's on the screen and don't pay attention to how much you're eating.

+ Get creative. There are many exercises you can do while watching TV. Here are a few examples:
  → Walk "laps" around the living room
  → Walk or run on a treadmill
  → Ride on a stationary bike
  → March in place
  → Do strength and flexibility exercises
  → Use exercise bands
  → Lift weights
  → Dance

+ Take breaks. If you're watching a longer program, exercise during the program and take recovery breaks during the commercials, or vice versa if you're very new to exercise.

+ Record your favorite shows. If you're pinched for time, record programs and skip through the commercials when you watch them later on. This can reduce watching time by about one-third.

+ Hide the computer or iPad. It's easy to click on the computer or iPad when it's right in front of you. Place the devices out of sight. "Out of sight, out of mind."

+ Be aware of cellphone use. You use your phone for many things, such as calling people or getting email. However, all of the social media outlets on your cellphone can become a mindless waste of time and keep you from doing other things. Limit unproductive time spent on your phone.

+ Find alternatives. Skip the screens altogether and go outside for a walk or bike ride or to do some yardwork. Seek out opportunities that help you break the habit of too much screen time.

YES, I CAN!

Use positive self-talk — "I can do this!" instead of "I can't do this." Talk yourself up, not down. Focus on positives, not negatives.

+ Put on some music. You're likely to move more if you listen to the radio. Another option is to listen to books on tape while working around the house.

+ Set up a screen zone. Set aside one place in the house to watch TV or use your computer or iPad. In particular, TV sets located in bedrooms and kitchens can lure you into motionless watching.

BREAK 2

No sugar

only what's naturally found in fruit

What:
If you want something sweet, eat fresh fruit. Otherwise, no sugar from common sources — candy, table sugar, brown sugar, honey, jam, jelly, desserts, sweets, and foods that contain more than a tiny amount of sugar or high-fructose corn syrup (such as soda and some coffee drinks).

Why:
Here are four key reasons why you should avoid sugar: 1. It contains calories. 2. It has no nutritional value. 3. If you're eating sugar, you're not eating something else that's healthier. 4. Sugar has direct negative health effects, such as tooth decay and an increase in blood sugar (glucose) associated with diabetes.

+ Clean out the cupboards. Before you start the program, rid your home of sweets and sodas, stock up on fresh fruit, and replenish the fruit regularly.

+ Read labels. Many products contain sugar. If corn syrup, dextrose, sucrose, glucose, fructose, maltose, turbinado, molasses or high-fructose corn syrup is listed among the first few ingredients on a label, the product likely has a high sugar content. Get rid of it.

+ Hide the wine and beer glasses. Alcohol is counted as a sugar, and no alcohol is allowed in the two-week *Lose It!* phase.

+ Sweeten with fruit. Instead of sugar or syrup, put fresh fruit on your morning cereal, oatmeal or pancakes. Also, avoid breakfast cereals that contain sugar.

+ Try different spices. Mix cinnamon with unsweetened applesauce as a spread on pancakes or toast. Other spices that may add sweetness include allspice, cardamom, cloves, ginger and nutmeg.

+ Experiment with naturally sweet drinks. Instead of soda, mix fruit juice with sparkling water.

- Enjoy fruit smoothies. Blend fresh fruit with fat-free vanilla frozen yogurt and some fruit juice and ice for a refreshing and naturally sweet treat.

- Test your culinary skills. For dessert, prepare baked apples or grilled pineapple.

- Be courageous. Use this two-week phase to experiment with new foods. Buy fruits such as kumquat, litchi, mango, papaya, pomegranate or star fruit, which can be obtained at many grocery stores or specialty food stores. Look for other foods that are naturally sweet to help soothe your sweet tooth.

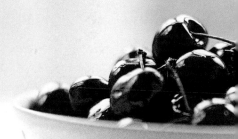

What about artificial sweeteners?

Why not just buy foods containing low-calorie artificial sweeteners? Sounds like a perfect solution. You get the sweetness of sugar without all the calories or carbohydrates. Not so fast!

Many ready-to-eat foods using low-calorie sweeteners — such as diet sodas, candies and cookies — have little nutritional value and should be avoided. In addition, studies have raised concerns that consuming foods containing low-calorie sweeteners may actually lead to increased calorie intake and weight gain (they may trick your brain into eating sweets at other times). Low-calorie sweeteners can be part of a healthy-eating plan — if they're used with care and in moderation. But in the two-week *Lose It!* phase, avoid them.

BREAK 3

No snacks

except vegetables and fruits

What:

If you snack between meals, make it only vegetables or fruits and nothing else.

Why:

Common snacks typically have a lot of calories and little nutritional value. However, vegetables and fruits are just the opposite — they can fill you up without contributing many calories to your daily total, and they're loaded with many healthy nutrients. Snacking on vegetables and fruits a couple of times a day can help you manage your weight, while snacking on most conventional commercial snacks can pack on pounds.

+ Clear out the cupboards. Before you start the program, remove from your home cookies, chips, candy, ice cream, and so on. Don't tuck them away in the back of a cupboard or freezer. Don't think you can resist the temptation to open the package. Get rid of them! If it's in your house, it's in your mouth.

+ Stock up. Instead of snacks, load up on plenty of ready-to-eat vegetables and fruits. Don't expect to get by with only apples or baby carrots. They should be two of many different options you can choose from. Think kiwi, mango, Bing cherries, sugar snap peas and sweet pepper slices.

+ Don't forget the office. Keep vegetables and fruits available at the office, too, so they're handy when you get hungry.

+ Eat regular meals. Establish a pattern of eating three meals every day. Space meals at intervals that are not too long. Allowing too much time to pass between meals can create a ravenous hunger that drives you to mindless snacking.

+ Sprinkle and dip. Experiment with different spices and herbs on vegetables and fruits to create new flavors. Another option is to dip them in fat-free yogurt or hummus.

+ Freeze it. Freeze fruits, such as grapes, for a cool and refreshing snack. Or make your own fruit ice pop by blending one or more fruits with a little juice and freezing the mixture.

+ Be proactive. Identify situations that lead you to snacking, and then try to avoid them or find alternate activities. If you habitually snack during work breaks, try going for a walk instead. If you can't resist a candy bar whenever you walk by the vending machine, try to avoid the vending machine. If emotions such as anger or sadness drive you to ice-cream cravings, talk to a friend who can listen and help relieve your urge to snack.

+ Be honest. Sometimes we snack not because we're hungry but as a way to relieve boredom or stress. As you reach for that snack, ask yourself if you're really hungry or just bored. If you're bored, find something else to do.

+ Distract yourself. Instead of having a snack, do something you enjoy. Exer-

The ice-cream parlor. The bakery. The food court at the mall. It may be hard to resist some of your favorite snacks when you can see — or smell — them. Remind yourself of how well you've done so far, and tell yourself that two weeks really isn't that long. And then keep on walking. Don't stop!

cise is an easy method of diverting your attention, but you can also work on a hobby, read a book, or call a family member or friend to visit.

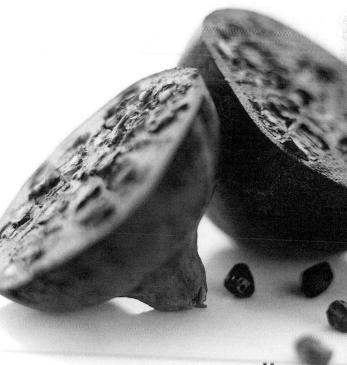

BREAK 4

Limited meat & low-fat dairy

the size of a deck of cards and low-fat dairy

What:
Picture the size of a deck of cards. Limit your total daily consumption of meat, poultry and fish to that (about 3 ounces of meat). In addition, if you consume dairy products, use only skim milk and low-fat products, and consume them in moderation.

Why:
All meat, even lean cuts and skinless poultry, have some saturated fat and cholesterol and can be high in calories. Plus, red meat and processed meats are associated with increased cancer risks. Full-fat dairy products also contain saturated fat that raises cholesterol. Alternatives that are lower in fat and calories are available for both meat and full-fat dairy products.

+ Don't make meat the focus. When planning your meals, make vegetables, fruits, whole-grain rice or pasta the main focus. Think of meat as a side to complement the other food items.

+ Think prime. When you do have meat, go for quality instead of quantity. Instead of a large piece of medium-quality meat, have a small piece of a good-quality cut.

+ Get rid of the fat. Trim all visible fat from meat sources, and remove the skin from poultry before preparing it.

+ Say goodbye to frying. Roast, broil, bake or grill your meat rather than frying it. The manner in which food is prepared greatly affects the amount of fat and calories you consume.

+ Eat more fish. At least two servings of fish are recommended each week. Along with being lower in saturated fat than is meat, fish — especially albacore tuna, salmon, mackerel and herring — is high in omega-3 fatty acids that reduce your risk of cardiovascular disease.

+ Go for the turkey. Substitute ground turkey for ground beef. When buying ground turkey, buy packages marked "ground turkey breast" versus "ground turkey," which may have the skin added.

+ Look for plant alternatives. Instead of meat as your daily source of protein, experiment with legumes and soy products, which are excellent alternatives to animal protein. A ½-cup serving of cooked beans, peas, lentils or tofu is about the same as a 2-ounce serving of meat, poultry or fish.

+ Go meatless more often. Experiment with a meatless meal at least once a week. Try eggplant lasagna or vegetable stir-fry dishes. Replace the meat in casseroles and sandwiches with fresh-cut or roasted vegetables. Enjoy a vegetable pizza with onions, peppers, mushrooms, tomato slices and artichokes. You can also make a meal of red beans and rice, split pea or lentil soups, or meatless three-bean chili (with kidney, black and garbanzo beans).

+ Look for *skim, low* and *reduced.* When buying and eating dairy products, avoid full-fat versions. Drink skim milk and buy low-fat yogurt and low-fat or reduced-fat cheese and cheese products.

Throughout the day, you'll make decisions that affect how well you follow this program. "Do I eat a hamburger and fries or a salad?" "Do I go for a walk or not?"

Be prepared for those moments of decision and strategize how best to guide yourself into making the right choice. Pretty soon those moments of decision will simply become habit.

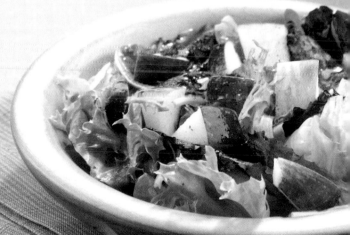

BREAK 5

No eating at restaurants

unless the meal fits the program

What:

Either don't eat out, or if you do, make sure you order foods and beverages that fit the habits in *Lose It!*

Why:

Eating out is associated with weight gain. The tantalizing sights and smells of a restaurant, deli counter, bakery display, food court or concession stand entice you with high-calorie menu items, often at times when you're not really hungry. The outcome is usually consuming far too many calories. In addition, most — if not all — restaurants serve large portions. And because the food is in front of you, you eat it.

+ Think fast. If you eat out because time is an issue, find recipes for easy-to-prepare — and healthy — meals you can quickly make at home. Do some of the prep work on weekends, so during the week you just have to assemble everything.

+ Stock up on staples. Make sure you have staple ingredients on hand to make basic dishes that you can prepare in a hurry. (See page 175 for a list of staples.)

+ Buy prepackaged. It's OK to buy fruits and veggies that are already cut, fish or chicken that's seasoned (but not breaded) and ready to go in the oven, or to pick up a healthy salad from the local deli on your way home.

If you do eat out:

+ Plan ahead. Adjust your day if you know you're going out to eat. For example, you might have a lighter lunch if you're eating supper at a restaurant. You might also schedule extra exercise time.

+ Eat first. Don't go to a restaurant famished. You'll eat more than you want, and you may not make the best meal choices. Have a healthy snack beforehand.

- Skip the appetizers. They often aren't the healthiest items on the menu, and they tend to be a source of hidden calories. If you have an appetizer, have vegetables or fruit.

- Salad or soup? Avoid cream-based soups and chowders. Broth-based vegetable soups are generally healthy. If you have a salad, request a plain vegetable salad with a low-fat dressing. Be wary of salad bars. Not all of the items are healthy, and it's easy to take more food than you need.

- Seek out something healthy. Fish or chicken are often the best options. Make sure vegetables are a prominent part of your meal. Choose steamed vegetables, a baked potato, boiled new potatoes, brown or wild rice, or fresh fruit instead of french fries, potato chips or mayonnaise-based salads.

- Speak up. Don't hesitate to make special requests. Most restaurants will honor them.

- Skip dessert. Unless there's something healthy on the menu, such as fresh fruit, shorbet or frozen yogurt, the best plan of action is to pass on dessert.

It can be very difficult going into a restaurant and not being able to order your favorite food. You may even feel like throwing in the towel. Don't!

Don't let giving up become an option. Instead, savor the experience, the atmosphere and the healthy food choice that you do make. Enjoy what you have instead of wishing for what you don't!

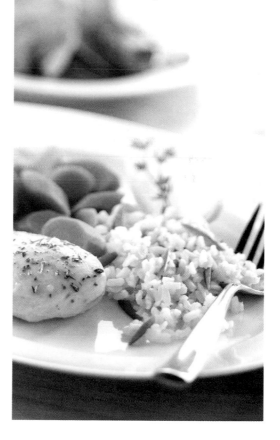

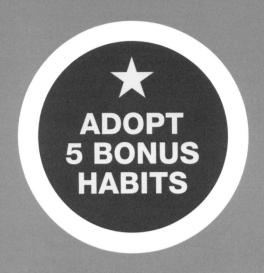

Chapter 4
Adopt
5 Bonus Habits

The Add 5 Habits and Break 5 Habits in *Lose It!* are must-dos. The 5 Bonus Habits here aren't must-dos but are recommended. They're all associated with weight loss. The more of them you follow — and the more closely you follow them — the more successful you're likely to be in your weight-loss efforts.

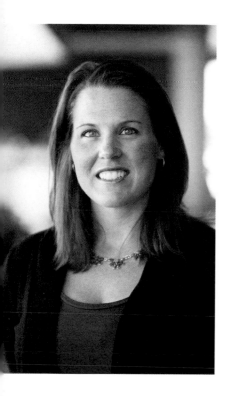

Sara M. Link
Mayo Clinic
Healthy Living Program

As a certified wellness coach, each day I work with individuals looking to make positive lifestyle changes. Being able to form new, healthy habits is key to their long-term success. This chapter gives you five bonus habits that can play key roles in your wellness journey.

Having to track your daily activities and everything you eat may seem overwhelming and tedious, but it can help you identify patterns of unhealthy behavior. And research shows that people who track both their food intake and activity level are generally more successful at achieving their weight-loss goals. Part of the reason may be that people tend to overestimate the amount of calories they burn and underestimate how many calories they consume.

Also, don't be frightened by the recommendation to move more. If time is a limiting factor, add extra movement into your daily routine. This might be as simple as using the restroom that's farthest away or standing and walking while you talk on the phone.

You may not know what approach will work best for you until you do a little experimentation. If one method doesn't work, try a different one. Keep at it, and you'll find a method that fits your lifestyle and can help you achieve long-term success.

Small daily changes become habits. Those habits become a routine, and eventually that routine becomes your lifestyle. What small changes will you make today?

BONUS 1

Keep food records

track everything you eat

What:
Keep a record of everything you eat and drink throughout the day, including types of food and the amounts. **JOT IT** ▸

Why:
Record keeping lets you know exactly what and how much you're eating. It also allows you to identify problem patterns in your eating behavior. People who keep food records are more successful at weight loss. You can use *The Mayo Clinic Diet Journal* to track what you eat. Or you can find an app for your cellphone or use an online food record. Even a notebook is fine if that works for you.

+ Make a log. Use some type of tracking tool to write down *everything* you eat. And *everything* means *everything*. **JOT IT** ▸

+ Indicate serving sizes. You will need to estimate food amounts in different measures. For fresh vegetables or fruits, list the size (small, medium or large). For pasta, rice, soups and beverages, indicate the number of cups or spoons. For baked goods, use approximate dimensions. For meat, poultry and fish, use approximate weight or size. See pages 256-283 for more on serving sizes.

+ Estimate. For mixed entrees such as casseroles or soup, do the best you can. Try to list the main ingredients.

+ Don't forget the extras. Pay attention to spreads, gravies and condiments that may accompany a food item. These items may have the most calories of anything you eat.

+ Snacks count too. Record snacks and other small items. They can add up!

+ So do fluids. Write down all beverages you drink, including the types (water, milk, juice, coffee) and how much you drink.

+ Keep it with you. Carry your journal with you at all times, so you can write down what you've eaten right away, and you don't have to try to remember later.

If you're unhappy with how your weight makes you look, take a photo of yourself, keep it with you, and look at it when you're facing a challenge. Tell yourself, "I'm making progress, and I'm not going back to looking like this!"

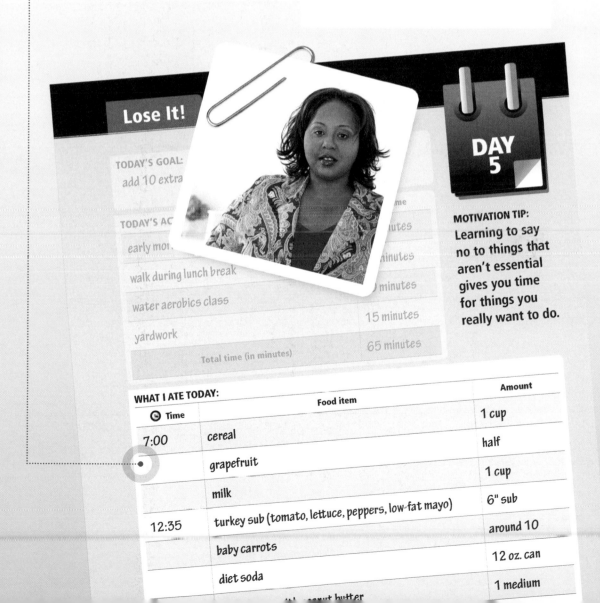

Lose It!

TODAY'S GOAL:
add 10 extra

TODAY'S AC

early mor...   ...utes

walk during lunch break   ...inutes

water aerobics class   ...minutes

yardwork   15 minutes

Total time (in minutes)   65 minutes

DAY 5

MOTIVATION TIP:
Learning to say no to things that aren't essential gives you time for things you really want to do.

WHAT I ATE TODAY:		Amount
⏱ Time	Food item	
7:00	cereal	1 cup
	grapefruit	half
	milk	1 cup
12:35	turkey sub (tomato, lettuce, peppers, low-fat mayo)	6" sub
	baby carrots	around 10
	diet soda	12 oz. can
	...nut butter	1 medium

BONUS 2

Keep activity records

track activity, duration and intensity

What:
Record all your exercise and physical activity throughout the day, including the type and duration. ▌**JOT IT** ▶

Why:
Record keeping helps you track the variety of activities and exercises that make up your day. Keeping a daily activity record for at least two weeks helps you to be accountable and should help you establish a regular exercise routine. Seeing your progress can build confidence and inspire you to set higher goals. Similar to your food record, there are various ways you can log this information. *The Mayo Clinic Diet Journal* **is one option.**

+ Five or more. Enter those activities that last five minutes or longer. This includes household chores, hobbies, recreational activities and exercise. Indicate the total amount of time for each activity. ▌**JOT IT** ▶

+ Note the intensity. Be aware of how intense an activity feels to you at the time you're doing it. Indicators are your heart rate, your breathing rate, perspiration and muscle fatigue. Take note of how slow or fast you performed each activity.

+ Note the distance. If you're walking or jogging, estimate the approximate distance you covered or the time you spent doing it. You may find it helpful to carry a watch or pedometer for this purpose.

+ Include other information. You might make note of weather conditions, the type of terrain, how you felt and whatever else you feel is important.

+ Take it slow. Don't become an overachiever because you feel pressure to fill up your activity record. The record should reflect reasonable (and achievable) exercise goals that you've set for yourself. Do what's safe and comfortable, even if that may mean leaving a few blank lines in your record.

+ Keep it handy. Similar to your food record, keep your activity record with you at all times. Write down what you did immediately afterward instead of trying to remember at the end of the day everything you did during the day.

+ Estimate. If you forgot to log something, do the best you can to remember what it was and for how long you did it.

RD · DAY 6

Lose It!

DAILY RECORD · DAY 5

DAY 5

TODAY'S GOAL:
add 10 extra minutes of exercise to my walking routine!

TODAY'S ACTIVITIES:

	⏲ Time
early morning walk	10 minutes
walk during lunch break	10 minutes
water aerobics class	30 minutes
yardwork	15 minutes
Total time (in minutes)	65 minutes

MOTIVATION TIP:
Learning to say no to things that aren't essential gives you time for things you really want to do.

WHAT I ATE TODAY:

BONUS 3

Move more!

walk or exercise for 60 minutes or more every day

What:
Increase your walking or exercise to 60 minutes or more every day. This doesn't have to be 60 minutes in addition to the 30 minutes or more in the earlier habit, Move! It's 60 minutes or more total. Of course, the more the better, within reason.

Why:
Increasing your physical activity to at least 60 minutes each day burns more calories and increases the health benefits you receive.

+ Follow this order: Increase the frequency, duration and intensity of your walking or exercise. The table on page 214 shows how to gradually increase the frequency and duration of a walking program. There are several ways to vary walking intensity, for example, by lengthening your stride, swinging your arms more, increasing your speed or walking up hills.

+ Take it slow. If you've been inactive for a while, be cautious with a 60-minute workout. Be sure to warm up and start slowly. Initially, it's enough that you're doing something daily. Your health and safety are the highest priority.

+ Start low. Keep the intensity low enough that you can quickly build up to 30 minutes throughout the day or at a time. Once you're comfortable with a longer duration, increase the intensity. Eventually try to increase to 60 minutes or more a day, and then once again increase the intensity of your activity.

+ Know your limitations. Take into account any medical or physical limitations in determining what's appropriate for you to do, but don't let lack of time or not wanting to change be an excuse for not exercising.

+ Schedule it. On your calendar, schedule time to exercise, just as you do meetings and appointments. You're more likely to exercise if it's on your calendar. It's one of the most important things you can do in your day.

+ Use a pedometer. Record how many steps you take each day for three consecutive days. Add the daily totals and divide by three to calculate your average number of steps each day. Set a goal to increase this average by either 2,000 or 3,000 steps a day until you reach a total of 10,000 daily steps. **JOT IT** ▶

Look for excuses to exercise rather than excuses not to exercise. Get past the first five or 10 minutes and the rest becomes easier. And the more frequently you exercise, the more you'll want to exercise.

+ Be flexible. To prevent boredom, do a variety of activities rather than just one. You might rotate between walking, bicycling and yoga, with a dance or an aerobics class thrown in as well. You might also switch between early morning and late afternoon exercise times.

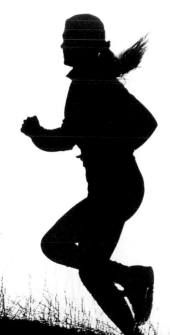

BONUS 4

Eat 'real food'

mostly fresh, and healthy frozen or canned food

What:
Eat only food that's in its natural state or is lightly processed — "real food." Limit or avoid more-processed foods, such as many canned and most boxed and convenience foods.

Why:
Food is processed to make it safe, available and convenient to use, but the processing may add unwanted fat, sugar, calories and salt. Real food is loaded with vitamins, minerals, fiber, antioxidants and other nutrients. Fast food is often filled with empty calories. Not everything that's processed is bad — but it's up to you to make the healthiest choices. Real food is often grown more locally and doesn't have as much packaging.

+ Plan ahead. You're more likely to eat real foods if you plan for them. When preparing your shopping list, make sure to include plenty of fresh fruits and vegetables. Then add whole-grain carbohydrates, such as brown rice and whole-grain pastas. Also include fish and lean meats.

+ Shop with purpose. Most real food is located in the produce and meat and seafood departments. When shopping, spend your time in these areas. Avoid aisles containing mostly processed items.

+ Make it lean. When purchasing proteins, such as fish, poultry and red meat, make sure you purchase lean varieties and limit the serving amount to the size of a deck of cards. These products should be in their natural state, not breaded, wrapped in bacon or marinated in a creamy sauce.

+ Frozen is fine. Freezing preserves the nutrients in vegetables and fruits, although the process may change their appearance slightly. Frozen vegetables and fruits can be quickly thawed and added to salads or other dishes.

+ Visit farmers markets. They are a great place to find fresh and great-tasting real foods.

+ Look at the label. If you do use prepared food products, read the Nutrition Facts label on the package. Choose foods with fewer calories and added ingredients. In general, the least processed ones have the shortest list of ingredients.

+ Rinse them. If you purchase canned vegetables, beans and legumes, rinse them in water to remove some of the excess sodium added during processing.

+ Keep it simple. Real foods often taste best when prepared simply so that their natural flavors come out. Look for simple menu ideas. These recipes also come in handy on days when plans change or you're feeling rushed.

+ Take advantage of prepackaged foods. Many groceries stock a variety of fresh vegetables and fruits that are packaged and ready for immediate use out of the bag. The stores may also package lean meats that have been trimmed and pre-cut for dishes such as stir-fries or kebabs.

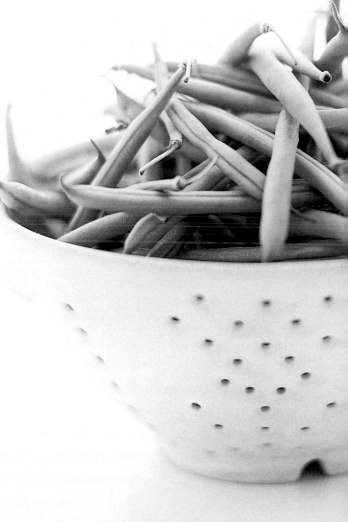

BONUS 5

Have a daily goal

something that motivates you

What:
Each day create a goal for yourself. It should be something that you can take action on and achieve during that day. Once you've determined your goal, write it down. **JOT IT** ▶

Why:
Your overall weight goal can often be met through a series of smaller performance goals that build on each other. Goal setting keeps you motivated and helps you stick with your program.

+ Place it front and center. Put your written goal where you can see it throughout the day. Read it several times a day to keep yourself motivated.

+ Don't make it weight related. Avoid daily goals based on weight loss, as your weight may vary from day to day due to fluid fluctuations in your body. When you achieve goals in activity and diet, weight loss should follow.

+ Be positive. Avoid resolute commands using "should," "must," "can't" or "won't." You subconsciously pick up on the negativity, which can lead to quick discouragement and failure. For example, rather than saying, "I won't eat junk food today," offer a solution such as, "When I'm hungry for a snack, I'll have some fruit."

+ Congratulate yourself. Make sure to give yourself a pat on the back when you reach your goal. Rewards are an important part of the process, whether it's the satisfaction of knowing that you did it or treating yourself to a simple foot massage or extra relaxation time.

+ Don't make it too easy. Setting a realistic goal doesn't mean it's an easy goal. It's true that there's danger in setting the bar too high. Nevertheless, you can judge a goal based on how it challenges your skills and resources — it should stretch them a little — and how committed you need to be — it should require some effort.

+ If at first you don't succeed. You may find yourself having to rephrase or rewrite a goal if you tried it and it didn't work. That's OK if you find the goal too challenging and you need to break it down. It's not OK if you're changing the goal simply out of convenience.

+ Look for other opportunities. In addition to a daily goal, before you go to bed you might jot down an inspirational message and tape it next to your bed or on the bathroom mirror, so it's the first thing you see in the morning. This message isn't meant to be a goal; rather its intent is to provide you with words of encouragement. A positive message right away in the morning may be just what you need to start your day on the right foot.

YES, I CAN!

Focus on today, not yesterday or tomorrow. Take it one day at a time, and your efforts will add up to success.

Just as in many aspects of life, when a goal is set for the future, it's easier for you to put it off — and it remains "for tomorrow." Rather than, "Tomorrow, I need to start walking more," write, "Today, I'm walking an extra 10 minutes."

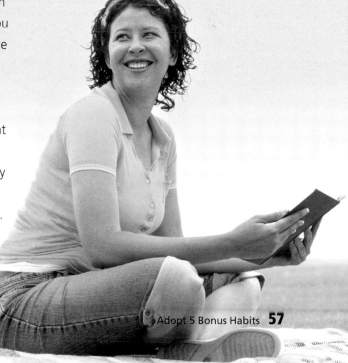

Chapter 5
What have you learned?

You're two weeks into a lifetime of better eating, moving more and enjoying a healthier weight. It's time to see what you can learn from what you've already done, so you can be even more successful in the future.

Congratulations! You've just completed *Lose It!*, the first two weeks of *The Mayo Clinic Diet*. Now it's time for a bit of reflection. How did these first two weeks go? Were they harder or easier than you anticipated?

Many people find the *Lose It!* phase isn't as difficult as it seems initially. In fact, you may have changed things you didn't think you could, which can be empowering.

Remember, the habits in *Lose It!* are "stretch goals." They're designed to bump you out of your comfort zone in a rather dramatic way and head you in a different direction. So give yourself a pat on the back for making it through.

Equally important, what did you learn from *Lose It!?* This is key because what you learned about yourself can help you be successful in the next phase of the diet, which is more long term.

As you analyze your *Lose It!* results, don't be too hard on yourself if you weren't perfect. That's OK. At this point, you're after patterns rather than

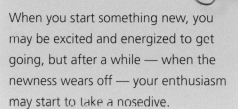

Staying motivated

When you start something new, you may be excited and energized to get going, but after a while — when the newness wears off — your enthusiasm may start to take a nosedive.

Losing weight is no different. Once this new journey you've embarked on loses some of its initial excitement, you may find yourself working harder to stay motivated.

That's why it's important to periodically take time to reconfirm your commitment to weight control. Review your reasons for wanting to shed some pounds, and remind yourself of the health benefits of doing so.

The longer you can keep on track, the easier it will be to stay on track!

perfection — eating more vegetables and fruits and less junk food, exercising more, and watching TV less. You get the picture.

Take what you learned from *Lose It!* and translate it into your personal plan for future success!

Analyzing your results

Lose It! is all about habits — changing old ones that contributed to your weight gain and adopting new ones that help you lose weight.

Analyzing your results from the two weeks of *Lose It!* can give you an idea of what was most effective in helping you establish or break these habits. (This review will also help if you decide to repeat *Lose It!* in the future.)

Note the emphasis on *you*. What works for someone else might not work for you, and vice versa.

Take a look at the habit trackers you filled out the past two weeks, as well as your daily goals, and the food and activity records you kept. **JOT IT** ▶

Use this information to identify personal patterns. If something worked well for you, why was that and how can you build on your success in the next phase of the diet?

If it didn't go so well, what were your obstacles? Is there a different approach that might work better?

1 Using your habit tracker, go across each row and add up the number of days that you followed each habit. Do each week individually, and then combine the totals for the two weeks. See an example of one week on the opposite page.

+ Which habits were strengths for you?

+ List some reasons why you did well on those habits.

+ Which habits didn't go as well?

+ List a few reasons why these habits were more challenging.

+ For those habits that were challenging, think of a couple of strategies for ways that you could do better. Check out the Action Guide on pages 234-255. It reviews common obstacles people face in trying to lose weight and strategies for overcoming them. Will any of the strategies work for you?

Habit tracker

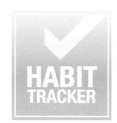

✔ **Check if done**

	Day 1	Day 2	Day 3	Day 4	Day 5	Day 6	Day 7	TOTALS
ADD 5 HABITS								
1. Eat a healthy breakfast	✔	✔		✔		✔	✔	5
2. Eat vegetables and fruits	✔	✔	✔		✔		✔	5
3. Eat whole grains	✔	✔	✔	✔		✔	✔	6
4. Eat healthy fats	✔	✔	✔	✔	✔		✔	6
5. Move!	✔		✔		✔	✔	✔	5
BREAK 5 HABITS								
1. No TV while eating			✔		✔		✔	3
2. No sugar	✔	✔	✔		✔	✔	✔	6
3. No snacks	✔	✔	✔	✔		✔	✔	6
4. Only moderate meat and dairy	✔	✔	✔	✔	✔		✔	6
5. No eating at restaurants	✔	✔	✔	✔	✔	✔		6
5 BONUS HABITS								
1. Keep diet records	✔	✔	✔	✔	✔	✔	✔	7
2. Keep exercise/activity records	✔	✔	✔	✔	✔	✔	✔	7
3. Move more!	✔						✔	2
4. Eat "real food"	✔	✔		✔			✔	4
5. Write your daily goals	✔	✔	✔	✔	✔	✔	✔	7
TOTALS:	14	12	12	10	10	9	14	

2 Using your habit tracker, add down each column and total up the number of habits you followed each day.

+ Which days of the week did you do better?

+ Are there reasons why you did better on certain days? Look at your journal or your daily goals to pick up clues.

+ If you didn't do well on certain days, what might be the reasons for that?

+ Again, can your daily journal or daily goals provide any clues? Look for patterns that may help you. Do you do better at the beginning of the week but lose momentum by the end of the week? Is there a particular day of the week that seems to pose a challenge?

+ As you did when evaluating each individual habit, page through the Action Guide to see if there may be a way to overcome what appears to be an obstacle.

3 Go to your weight record in *The Mayo Clinic Diet Journal* (or in a notebook or on your phone) where you kept track of your weight. Add up the amount of weight you lost. Also measure your waist.

+ Did you lose more weight in one week than in the other? If so, might there be a reason for that?

+ Did your waist size decrease? If so, how much? Muscle gained through increased physical activity may decrease your waist measurement.

+ Does what you learned from evaluating your habits coincide in any way to changes in your weight?

4 While it's important, don't get too caught up in the analysis. You probably have a pretty good idea why some changes went well and others didn't. Take what you learned, and let's move on. It's time to begin the next phase!

What's the real reason?

As you analyze your habit tracker and other daily records, think about the last two weeks and what you might have learned about yourself and your habits. For example, if weekends are more difficult for you to follow a healthy diet and exercise, why is that?

Often, there's more to the story ...

+ Do I eat when I'm bored, anxious or stressed?

+ Is it harder for me to maintain good habits in certain places — at home, at the mall, at the office?

+ Am I better at following the diet when I'm with others and not by myself?

+ Do I spend too much time in front of screens — phone, computer, and TV?

+ When I'm relaxing instead of working, do I tend to put off things that I should be doing until it's too late?

As you transition into *Live It!*, perhaps your biggest challenge will be keeping yourself from sliding back into old habits. As you go through *Live It!*, occasionally revisit the pages of *Lose It!* to help keep yourself on track.

Now, on to *Live It!*

Part 2 *Live It!*

Lose It! gave you a quick start. **Live It!** puts you on a path you can enjoy for a lifetime.

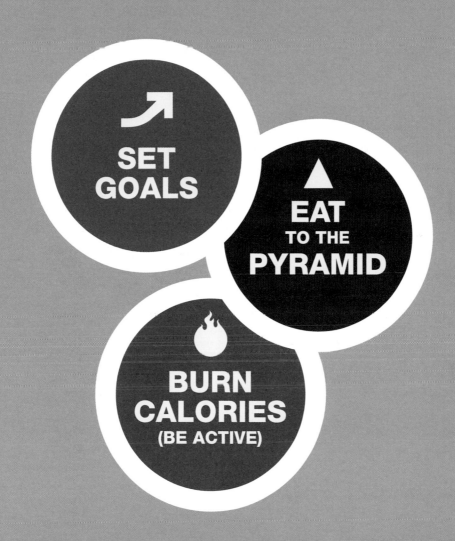

SET GOALS

EAT TO THE PYRAMID

BURN CALORIES (BE ACTIVE)

It's transition time. Let's go!

Chapter 6
The next phase

Lose It! is a bit like learning how to swim by being tossed in the pool and doing whatever it takes to keep your head above water. It's not very subtle or refined, but the results are immediate. Now that you know how to dog paddle, *Live It!* gives you the tools and techniques to help you swim the distance!

Congratulations! You've made it through the *Lose It!* phase. Give yourself a big pat on the back. Sure, you may not have done things perfectly every single day. Maybe you had a doughnut one morning at work. Or maybe you hunkered down in front of the TV last Saturday and never got to the gym like you were supposed to. But all in all, you stuck to the habit changes on most days, even though it was challenging at times.

And that's the key. Perfection isn't the goal. Stick-to-it-iveness is. Ideally, what you've shown yourself is that change is possible — and not as hard as you initially believed. Not long ago, you couldn't have imagined an afternoon break without a candy bar and a soda. But now you've found that you don't mind clementines or unsweetened ice tea. Plus, you feel better.

The whole purpose of *Lose It!* was for you to jump in and change a number of habits that hopefully led to real weight loss. In general, the more habits people change, the more weight they lose. There weren't many details in *Lose It!*, such as how many

calories you should eat each day, and that was intentional. By changing key habits related to eating and exercise, you were able to lose weight without getting lost in the details. Hopefully, this empowered you and gave you added confidence.

Transitioning from *Lose It!* to *Live It!* is about staying on track and building on the changes you've made. Remember, over time, small, consistent changes can add up to big results.

Whenever you encounter everyday decisions — whether it's choosing between a cookie or an apple, a walk or a nap — *Live It!* is designed to consistently guide you toward the choice that helps you achieve your goals. Because, as you'll see, that's what this transition is all about — a turning point that marks a new way of caring for yourself, complete with a fresh mindset and limitless possibilities.

From short-term to lifelong

One of the key goals of *Lose It!* was to create a mental reset so that you're no longer tied to your old ways of thinking about eating and moving. Your job now is to start thinking in terms of a lifelong approach. While this book may be called *The Mayo Clinic Diet*, the word *diet* describes a sustainable eating pattern, not a diet that you go "on" and "off" of, in the popular sense of the word.

This new way of eating — and moving — is something you keep for life. And because it's based on a number of general principles, there are endless ways of staying with it without getting bored or overwhelmed.

So, what about the habits you've worked on so far? Yes, some of them may have been more challenging than others. While you may not be able to maintain all of the habits perfectly as time goes on, try to maintain as many of them as you can, and build on them.

The first five habits — *Adopt five habits* — are lifestyle strategies you want to keep for life. Maintain them as much as possible. Each day, eat a healthy breakfast, plenty of fruits and vegetables, whole grains and healthy fats, and make time for physical activity.

The second five habits — *Break five habits* — are intended to limit behaviors that add unnecessary calories. People often wonder whether these rules still need to be followed after the *Lose It!* phase. Yes, they do, as much as possible. But on occasion, it's OK to bend the rules a bit:

+ **Sugar.** Will you ever have a piece of dessert or a glass of wine again? Yes, you will. But the distinguishing factor is habitual versus occasional. Can you have cake on your birthday? Yes. Should you have cake or dessert every day? No. Keep sugar special and limit it.

+ **Restaurants.** No, we're not saying you can never eat at restaurants again. But try to eat at home more often because you tend to eat healthier when making your own meals.

+ **Snacks.** If you can make the switch on this one — keep processed snacks out of your house and stock your kitchen with fruits and veggies — eventually you won't think twice about grabbing a juicy peach or some sugar snap peas to satisfy a craving. What about the Super Bowl party at your friend's house? Go and have some (not all!) of the food, but keep the occasion special and return to your regular routine the next day.

+ **Screens.** The habit of eating while in front of a screen — TV, computer, cellphone — is best broken for good. This doesn't mean you can't have some unbuttered popcorn at the movies, but TV dinners should largely remain a thing of the past. If it works for you to exercise while watching TV, keep it up.

The last habits were the *Bonus habits*. Some of these habits you should strive to maintain for life — such as eating "real," not processed, food and exercising more often. When it comes to keeping records, continue the activity until you feel like you've got a handle on the big picture — you've learned your weaknesses and the triggers behind them.

Keep in mind that if you start gaining weight again and you aren't sure why, you can always restart your food and activity records.

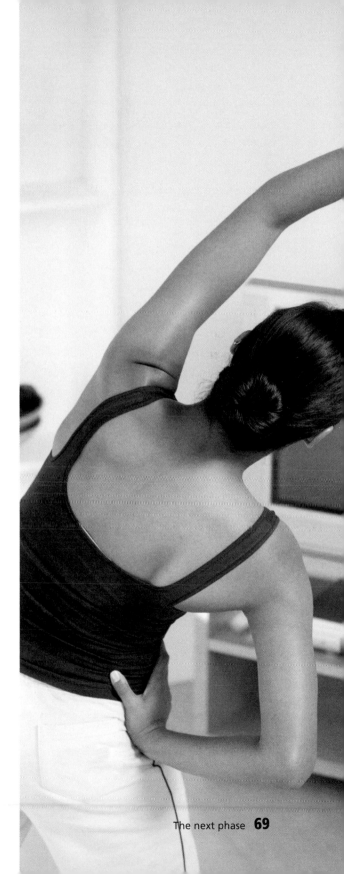

A new path

In the chapters ahead, you'll take a deep dive into *Live It!* You'll learn specific methods and strategies that will help you go the distance in your quest for a lifelong healthy weight. You'll set goals and determine your calorie limits. You'll learn what a food serving is and how many calories it contains just by looking at it. And you'll develop strategies for how to burn even more calories. You'll also find help and advice on shopping, creating menus, overcoming common obstacles, and maintaining your motivation.

Think of this as a journey in which you continue to make ongoing changes as time goes on. Soon, you may find yourself eating foods that you never thought you'd eat because you didn't like them — or thought you didn't. With the right attitude, you can learn to like new foods, and there are a lot of wonderful foods out there.

If you remain open and curious, the journey will only get better as you move forward. Here's a simple example. Say you start out eating a basic salad for lunch — lettuce, tomatoes, cucumbers, hard-boiled eggs, and a simple oil and vinegar dressing. But then you realize that baby spinach also makes a good salad. And what if you add some toasted sunflower seeds or some cooked quinoa? And wouldn't some red onions or roasted beets look nice with it? Soon enough, you'll have an expanding repertoire of salads only limited by the ingredients you have available and your imagination. You may even enjoy the challenge of using what's in season at the moment and seeing what you can come up with.

Yes, change can be challenging, but don't underestimate yourself. Look at what you accomplished in *Lose It!* Even if you only take very small steps in the beginning, as long as you keep moving down the path of healthy weight loss, the journey will become more enjoyable.

Is it really this easy? No, or everyone would be doing it. Is it possible? Absolutely, and you're on your way. Don't be surprised if you encounter some roadblocks ahead — everyone does. Specific chapters in this book can help you identify obstacles that may pop up and how to become your own best problem-solver. The Action Guide is filled with common problem scenarios people face and how to overcome them. Chapter 20 helps you deal with slip-ups and how to get back on track.

It's your life

Although you receive a lot of guidance in this book, keep in mind that this is your journey and your plan — not your mother's, not your best friend's, not your neighbor's. This is you forging your own path toward a healthier lifestyle.

Make the plan yours. Design it and tailor it in a way that fits you. Having a plan that's individualized to your tastes and lifestyle will make it easier to keep up over time. This individualized approach is much better than continuing to search for the elusive silver (weight-loss) bullet. This doesn't mean, however, that you can't or shouldn't reach out to others for support — family, friends, professionals (see Chapter 12).

As you learn the basic concepts of how to eat healthy and become more active, make sure the execution fits you — your schedule, priorities and overall philosophies. Weight loss is a complex process. There are literally hundreds of factors that affect weight and activity. Your job is to determine what you need to do to make your plan work for you. And don't feel you can't make changes along the way. If something isn't working, try another approach.

Also, keep it simple. Try not to get hung up on details, such as the precise number of food group servings in your meal or exactly how many calories you burned swimming those laps. You may have heard the saying, "Don't let the perfect be the enemy of the good." Sometimes, paying too much attention to the details can make it even more difficult to reach your goals.

Finally, feel free to revisit the two-week *Lose It!* phase anytime you need a refresher course or you feel yourself slipping back into old habits. Consider *Lose It!* your personal reset button that you can use at any time you feel you need to get back on track.

Eventually — as you become comfortable managing your diet and daily activities — you may leave this book behind. The goal of the book is to get you to a point where you're fully in control and you have the skills needed to maintain a healthy lifestyle. As your new eating and activity routines become second nature (they become habit!), you'll make decisions that will automatically default to the healthy option. You'll know what to do, on your own!

Live It! in real life

We are all different. That is why this next phase — *Live It!* — won't play out the same for everybody. Here are some different scenarios as to how the diet may work, depending on your life circumstances and individual preferences.

Shayla, age 44

Bio: Married, three school-age children, self-employed, owns small graphic-design business
Lifestyle: Busy working mom, not a lot of time for meal preparation, prefers to spend her free time with her family
Goals: Wants to lose some weight, have more energy, feel good about herself

6:00 a.m.	Rises, lets dog out, makes coffee, wakes rest of the family
6:15 a.m.	Eats breakfast: a plate of pre-cut fruit, whole-grain toast topped with almond butter, orange juice
7:00 a.m.	Walks children to bus stop; once children are off, takes the dog for a 30-minute walk
7:35 a.m.	Does 15-minute strength-training program; prepares for the day
8:30 a.m.	Works in home office; takes frequent stretch breaks
10:30 a.m.	Grabs some yogurt and a cup of tea for midmorning snack
12:30 p.m.	Prepares lunch: tomato, basil and tuna salad seasoned with salt, pepper and a dash of olive oil and lime juice, fresh berries, and water with lemon
1:30 p.m.	Parks the car and walks several blocks to meet with a client
3:30 p.m.	Puts out fresh veggies and hummus dip for a snack when kids get home from school
4:00 p.m.	Helps with homework; hangs out with kids
5:00 p.m.	Prepares shrimp and vegetable stir-fry with quick-cooking brown rice for dinner; eats with the family
6:15 p.m.	Does yoga with kids while watching TV, answers emails
8:00 p.m.	Prepares kids' school lunches
9:00 p.m.	Watches TV with husband and relaxes; has plain popcorn for a snack
10:00 p.m.	Gets ready for bed; reads
10:30 p.m.	Lights out

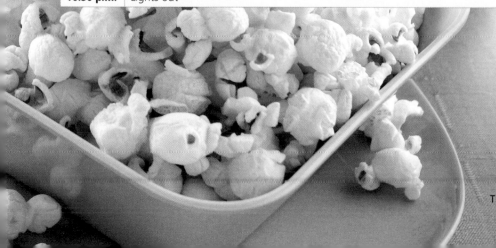

Steve, age 30

Bio: Single, legal counsel for pharmaceutical firm
Lifestyle: Works long hours, not a big breakfast eater,
likes to cook and appreciates nice restaurants
Goals: Wants to lose weight, become more fit, have more energy

6:30 a.m.	Rises; does a few stretches and strength and core exercises; gets ready for the day
7:00 a.m.	Prepares a breakfast smoothie with fresh fruit
7:30 a.m.	Drives to work; parks in a remote lot and walks several blocks to downtown office; grabs coffee and newspaper on the way
10:30 a.m.	Takes a break and walks around the office; refreshes coffee and grabs handful of plain roasted nuts from container in his desk
12:30 p.m.	Lunches with company clients; has grilled fish with a side salad and sparkling water
3:00 p.m.	Snacks on some plain popcorn
5:30 p.m.	Wraps up work and heads to the gym; does personalized workout and plays racquetball with a friend in a local league
6:30 p.m.	Heads home; listens to an audiobook in car
7:30 p.m.	Prepares dinner of wild rice pilaf with carrots and dried cherries, grilled chicken breast, arugula dressed with garlic and lemon juice
8:30 p.m.	Watches favorite TV show
9:30 p.m.	Surfs the web; reads or catches up with friends
10:30 p.m.	Gets ready for bed
11:00 p.m.	Lights out

Max and Jean, ages 60 and 62

Bio: Max works a split-shift schedule, Jean is retired, grandchildren visit often
Lifestyle: More free time on their hands, varying schedules, different food preferences
Goals: Want to stay healthy and fit for travel, keep up with their grandchildren, Jean wants to lose some weight

7:30 a.m.	Both rise; Max has oatmeal, banana and coffee for breakfast and Jean has yogurt with fruit and tea; prepare for day
10:00 a.m.	Go for a walk in the neighborhood park
11:00 a.m.	Shop, run errands
12:00 p.m.	Lunch at restaurant where Jean has a salad and Max has a club sandwich and coleslaw
1:15 p.m.	Max goes to work, brings healthy frozen entree for dinner; Jean does errands around the house
3:00 p.m.	Jean has a cup of tea and some fresh grapes
4:00 p.m.	Jean rides her stationary bike while watching an afternoon talk show
5:00 p.m.	Jean heats up leftovers from last night's dinner of chicken sausage meatballs and cauliflower mashed potatoes
6:00 p.m.	Jean video chats with her daughter and grandchildren
6:45 p.m.	Jean walks to weekly church meeting
9:00 p.m.	Max returns from work and Jean from her meeting; they relax, watch some TV and compare total steps on their fitness trackers; Max does lower back exercises recommended by his therapist; they each have a piece of toast with jelly
11:00 p.m.	Jean turns on some soothing music while getting ready for bed
11:30 p.m.	Lights out

Chapter 7
Know your goals

How much do you want to weigh? Chances are less than you do now or you wouldn't be reading this book. You may have a specific number in mind, but before you get your mind set on a certain weight, let's talk about personal goals and how they can help you be successful.

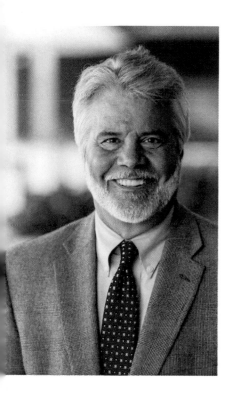

Philip T. Hagen, M.D.
Preventive Medicine

For people trying to lose weight, setting goals can often mean the difference between success and failure. Goals help motivate you and keep you focused. They put your thoughts into actions and help you meet your expectations.

But goal-setting isn't as easy as it may seem. You can't just write something down and expect that it will happen.

Your ability to reach your weight-loss goals is closely tied to how realistic they are. Many people have unrealistic expectations when it comes to weight loss. They set goals for themselves that are too big, too quick, too impractical.

Before you identify your goals, take some time to reflect on your situation. You know you want to lose weight, but why? Why is this so important to you? What is it that you're really striving for?

Once you have some answers (or at least some pretty good assumptions), develop your plan. Break those big goals down into smaller steps that seem within your grasp. The information in the pages that follow will show you how to do that.

Many people learn a lot about themselves in this process, and they're surprised by what they can achieve with the right attitude and a good plan!

Achieving and maintaining a healthy weight is a lifelong journey, and there may be times when the task may seem overwhelming. Losing weight is a big project — possibly one of your biggest undertakings yet.

As with any big project, if you focus only on the end result (which may seem endlessly far away!) the process may seem daunting. The key to achieving your ultimate goal is knowing how to break it down into smaller, achievable and realistic goals that build up to the final result.

Goals are essential to making any big change. They help you chart your course toward change and transform longings and dreams into practical, meaningful milestones.

This chapter provides a hands-on guide to help you establish and achieve your goals. In this chapter we'll talk about personal goals. In the next chapter we'll introduce pyramid targets. These are eating guidelines based on the Mayo Clinic Healthy Weight Pyramid (see page 32), designed to help you achieve your personal goals.

It's OK to dream big

Big things don't happen unless you have big aspirations. But recognize that big things typically don't happen without big efforts.

Champion athletes don't become champions and then start training like one. It's the other way around — they dream big, do the necessary preparation and then carry out their plan to reach their goals.

So dream big if you want to — keeping realism in mind — but understand that you'll need a well-planned effort to reach that weight loss goal.

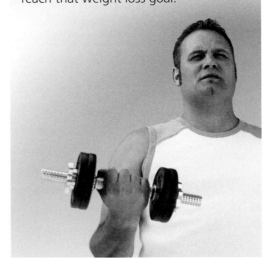

Personal goals

Your personal goals are those goals that you set for yourself. When you started the program a couple of weeks ago, you may have had some personal goals in mind. Losing weight is likely at the top of that list, but you may have also set goals for getting in better physical shape, adopting a healthier diet or just feeling better.

If you haven't already, write down each of your goals on a piece of paper. Underneath, write why this goal is important to you. What is it that's motivating you to make this big change? Would you like a better figure or to be able to fit into a smaller clothing size? Are you looking to reduce the amount of medication needed to control your blood pressure or cholesterol levels? You may have more than one motivator.

Ask yourself how important each goal is to you. In general, the more important a goal is, the more willing you may be to do what it takes to reach that goal. Realistically examining each of your goals can help prioritize them and identify where your efforts should be focused.

Now ask yourself how confident you are that you can achieve each of the goals you've written down? On a scale of 1 to 10, if your confidence level is below a 7, you may want to scale down your goal a bit to a target that you have confidence you can achieve. If you have more than one goal, consider whether working on multiple goals at once will be distracting or energizing.

Analyzing your goals may cause you to refine or even change them. Perhaps your goal of losing 50 pounds was sparked by your upcoming class reunion, but now you realize what you really want is just to get healthier and feel better.

Most often, personal goals tend to center around weight, activity, healthy eating and feeling better.

Weight goal

When it comes to setting a specific weight-loss goal, there's really no wrong answer as long as your goal weight is safe (healthy) and realistic. (Take a look at the body mass index chart on page 145 as a guide to reaching a healthy weight.)

What might a realistic goal be? Depending on your weight, 10 percent of your current weight might be a good start. That's 18 pounds if you weigh 180 pounds, or 25 pounds if you weigh 250 (and so on).

You don't have to try to reach your long-term weight goal right away. Your long-term weight goal may not be a realistic way to start. It may be easier if you break it up into smaller short-term goals. Depending on your weight, 5 percent of your current weight might be a good start. That's 9 pounds if you weigh 180 pounds, or 12.5 pounds if you weigh 250 pounds. Your doctor may be able to help you set a specific goal based on your health.

Activity goal

Just as there's no wrong answer in determining how many pounds you should lose, there's no specific amount of exercise you must do either. However, as a general goal, try to aim for at least 30 minutes of physical activity most days of the week. Remember, any and all activity helps, so long as it's healthy and safe.

As you likely know by now, being active is an integral component of long-term weight loss. Regular exercise leads to more and stronger muscles. And lean muscle mass burns more energy (calories) than fat does, which keeps you losing weight longer.

What physical activity goals did you set for yourself in the *Lose It!* phase, and how did they work for you? Is it time to amp it up a little now? Or did you bite off a little more than you can chew? It's good to challenge yourself, but you also want to set yourself up for success. Make sure the goals you set are ones you can reasonably achieve.

Healthy eating goal

Perhaps one of your goals is simply to eat better. There are many ways you can do this, and any change that you can make to improve your diet is good.

Performance vs. outcome

There are two types of goals that can help your weight-loss effort. You need them both to be successful:

+ **Outcome goals.** An outcome goal focuses on an end result. "I want to weigh 145 pounds," or "I want to lose 30 pounds."
+ **Performance goals.** A performance goal focuses on a process or action. "I will walk 30 minutes each day," or "I will eat four servings of vegetables each day."

Performance goals are the smaller steps that can help you achieve your big outcome goal. Setting an outcome goal without performance goals is like trying to run a marathon without training for it — you don't have much chance for success (and it's likely to be a painful experience).

An outcome goal becomes easier to achieve when it's coupled with performance goals that provide the steps necessary to get you to the desired outcome. Establishing small, everyday performance goals not only makes the process more doable, it also allows you more room to personalize and tweak your approach as you go along. Once you're able to do that, the whole endeavor becomes much more manageable, enjoyable and sustainable.

For weight loss, you don't necessarily need a big outcome goal. Some people find that just focusing on the process of eating well and moving more (using performance goals) is more effective than setting a larger outcome goal. Others find that aiming for a specific weight goal helps keep them motivated and on track.

Just remember, sometimes achieving a number of modest short-term goals is more effective than aiming for a bigger and less realistic outcome goal.

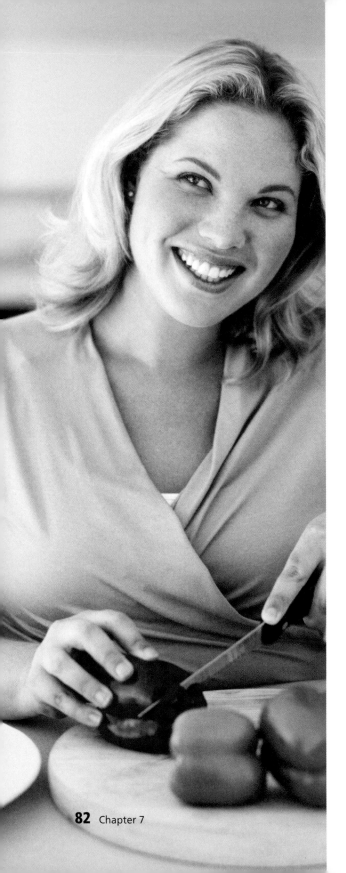

Think about what you see as your problem areas — your downfalls. What are some changes you can make to help fix these problems?

Maybe your goal is to eat less red meat and more fish or seafood, to munch on fruit when you're hungry instead of candy or chips, or to eat more vegetables with your meals. The list is endless.

In the two-week *Lose It!* phase, we asked you to make some specific dietary changes. Which of these changes can you continue to follow and build on? Which may take more time and patience? Consider these factors as you establish your goals.

Feeling better goal

Wouldn't it be nice to have more energy, move around easier and just feel good about yourself? It sure would, and you can easily make it happen. You can achieve your feel better goal by reaching your other goals. Working on your eating and activity goals will not only help you reach your weight goal, you'll also feel better.

Setting SMART goals

As you contemplate and prepare to jot down your personal goals, think about how you're going to achieve those goals. Your chances of success are much greater if you set performance goals that are SMART:

Specific. State exactly what you want to achieve, how you're going to do it and when you want to achieve it. For example, instead of saying, "I'm going to exercise more," say, "I'm going to walk for 15 minutes during my lunch hour every day."

Measurable. How will you know if you've reached your goal if you can't measure it? If your goal is to walk 15 minutes at lunch, wear a watch so that you'll know when you've walked that long. Or try an activity-tracking device, such as a fitness watch, to monitor how many steps you take in a day. How to measure and record your goals is discussed in Chapter 11.

JOT IT ▶

Attainable. Set a goal that is realistic and that you have sufficient time and resources to achieve. If anything, err on the side of starting off too easily. It's better to succeed at one small change and increase your goal for next week than to try too much, fail and give up.

Relevant. Set a goal that's important and that means something to you. It doesn't have to be huge and lofty to be relevant.

Time-limited. You should be able to complete your goal in a timely manner. Being able to track your progress, as mentioned earlier, not only keeps you motivated but helps ensure that you complete your goal within a set time frame.

Once you've identified your goals, place them somewhere that you can see them. Don't shove them in a drawer or keep them hidden in your journal. Out of sight, out of mind!

Check in often to monitor how you're progressing. Are the goals you've set too easy, too difficult or about right? Don't be afraid to make changes as you go along. Be focused, yet flexible.

Chapter 8
Set your targets

If you don't like to count calories, you're in luck — you don't have to! In this chapter, you'll learn how you can keep your daily calorie level within a "close enough" range so that you can lose weight without having to keep track of the calories in each item you eat.

Now come the specifics — the daily nitty-gritty of how to turn some of your personal goals into reality. During the first two weeks of the diet, we set forth some general concepts to help you lose weight — basically, eat more of this and less of that.

In the *Live It!* phase, we offer a more specific plan for how many calories you should consume each day to lose weight, and what foods you should eat to help you stay within that calorie limit. We do this by setting pyramid targets. The food choices in these targets are based on the Mayo Clinic Healthy Weight Pyramid, which is basically your playbook for healthy eating.

The pyramid targets serve two purposes. First, they can help you lose weight so that you reach your weight goal. Equally, if not more, important, they'll help you maintain your weight loss by establishing a healthy eating program that you can enjoy for a lifetime.

Basically, the targets teach you how to eat healthy. And after doing it long enough, it becomes habit.

Selecting your daily calorie target

To get started on your eating plan, first up is to determine your daily calorie target. To lose weight, you need to take in fewer calories than what you're currently consuming. To do this, it helps to set a target.

In the *Live It!* phase, your goal is to lose about 1 to 2 pounds a week. That means consuming at least 500 to 1,000 calories a day less than you normally do. If you eat 500 fewer calories each day than normal and you keep your activity level about the same, you should lose about 1 pound in a week. That's because 3,500 calories equals about a pound of body fat.

You can go through the process of tracking how many calories you consume over a week, averaging that number and then subtracting 500 to 1,000 calories to determine your target, but that's a lot of work and not really necessary. We've simplified things with the table on the next page, which is based on average calorie intakes needed to lose 1 to 2 pounds a week.

Your daily calorie target for healthy weight loss

Weight in pounds	Starting calorie target			
Women	**1,200**	**1,400**	**1,600**	**1,800**
250 or less	✔			
251 to 300		✔		
301 or more			✔	
Men	**1,200**	**1,400**	**1,600**	**1,800**
250 or less		✔		
251 to 300			✔	
301 or more				✔

On the chart above, find your current weight and the calorie target associated with that weight. This is a good place to start.

You can adjust the target based on your own goals and how quickly you want to lose weight. If you feel exceptionally hungry or lose weight too quickly, consider moving up to the next calorie level. If you're moving down a calorie level, don't drop below the lowest level listed. Fewer than 1,200 daily calories for women and 1,400 for men generally aren't recommended because you may not get enough nutrients.

Determining your daily servings targets

Now you know how many calories you should consume in a day, but the thing is, you don't eat calories, you eat food. Again, you can go through some pretty detailed tracking and analysis to convert the food you eat into calories, but that can be a lot of work. To simplify things, this program focuses on servings from food groups in the Mayo Clinic Healthy Weight Pyramid rather than on calories.

Using your daily calorie target, look at the table on the next page to

Serving recommendations for daily calorie targets

Food group	Daily calorie targets				
	1,200	**1,400**	**1,600**	**1,800**	**2,000**
V Vegetables	4 or more	4 or more	5 or more	5 or more	5 or more
F Fruits	3 or more	4 or more	5 or more	5 or more	5 or more
C Carbohydrates	4	5	6	7	8
PD Protein/Dairy	3	4	5	6	7
Ft Fats	3	3	3	4	5

determine how many servings from the pyramid food groups you should eat each day. Tracking servings is a lot easier than counting calories, and it gives a "close-enough" measurement of calorie intake. It also provides a guide to what kind of foods to eat, ensuring that you get a balanced diet.

Note that the servings listed for the carbohydrates, protein/dairy and fats groups are upper limits. Try not to exceed them. No one is perfect, but the closer you stick to the targets for these food groups, the more likely you are to be successful in losing weight.

Vegetables and fruits are a little different. The servings targets for these food groups are lower limits. We want you to eat at least the number of servings listed, and you can eat more if you want to.

Now, don't freak out when you see you'll be eating at least four servings of vegetables a day and three servings of fruit. As you'll see in the pages that follow, what you think of as a serving may not be all that much. And, we'll give you plenty of tips along the way to help you meet your targets.

Eating this many servings of vegetables and fruits is not something most people are used to. But studies show that eating more vegetables and fruits is a key factor in weight management.

A portion vs. a serving

Your first reaction to seeing how many servings of some foods you'll be eating with this diet might have been, "I can't do that!" Hold on — you may be confusing servings with portions.

The Mayo Clinic Healthy Weight Pyramid defines a serving as an exact amount of food, based on common measurements such as cups, ounces and tablespoons. Don't confuse a serving with a portion. A portion is the amount of food you put on your plate. A portion of food may contain several servings.

One of the reasons more people today are overweight or obese is that portion sizes have increased, especially in restaurants. We've become accustomed to eating large amounts of food at our meals — far more than we need!

To lose weight, and keep it off, you need to learn how to estimate servings so that you can control portions. Throughout the book, we provide a number of tools and tips to help you do that.

Serving sizes at a glance

Your task going forward is to be able to look at different foods and quickly estimate how much equals one serving. It may sound difficult, but it's not. That's because we provide you with methods to calculate serving sizes.

On the opposite page is a chart that offers visual cues to help you gauge Mayo Clinic Healthy Weight Pyramid servings for the various food groups.

Keeping these visual cues in mind, you can construct meals to meet your servings recommendations. For example, the chicken breast you have for dinner should be about the size of a deck of cards, half a baked potato about the size of a hockey puck, the butter you put on top of the potato about the size of one die, the carrots to go with the chicken about the size of a baseball, and your diced pineapple about the size of a tennis ball.

Using these visual cues will get you "close enough" to actual servings. On pages 256-283 you can find specific serving sizes for various foods.

Quick guide to serving sizes

Vegetables	Calories	Visual cue
1 cup broccoli	25	1 baseball
2 cups raw, leafy greens	25	2 baseballs

Fruits	Calories	Visual cue
½ cup sliced fruit	60	Tennis ball
1 small apple or medium orange	60	Tennis ball

Carbohydrates	Calories	Visual cue
½ cup pasta or dried cereal	70	Hockey puck
½ bagel	70	Hockey puck
1 slice whole-grain bread	70	Hockey puck
½ medium baked potato	70	Hockey puck

Protein/Dairy	Calories	Visual cue
3 ounces of fish	110	Deck of cards
2-2½ ounces of meat	110	⅔ deck of cards
1½-2 ounces of hard cheese	110	⅓ deck of cards

Fats	Calories	Visual cue
1½ teaspoons peanut butter	45	2 dice
1 teaspoon butter or margarine	45	1 die

These visual cues can help you use the food lists that begin on page 256.

Making sense of servings

Estimating your servings at meals is a great way to control the calories you consume. Unfortunately, the eye can be deceiving. Most people habitually, and unintentionally, underestimate the number of servings they eat. This means they consume more calories than they think they're getting, and they can't understand why they're gaining weight. Here's an exercise to help you get a better sense of servings.

Pour dry cereal into a bowl until you have what you think is about ½ cup. Don't use a measuring device; just depend on your own estimation.

Now pour the cereal out of the bowl and into a measuring cup. How close did you come to ½ cup? If you overestimated, don't feel discouraged. Most people imagine ½ cup being a greater amount than it actually is. Try this exercise again to see if you can get a closer estimate. One serving of most dry cereal is the equivalent of ½ cup.

You can try this same exercise the next time you're cooking pasta. After you've drained the cooked pasta, place what you think is a serving onto your plate, then put it into a measuring cup. One serving of cooked pasta is about ½ cup. How did you do?

Try this exercise with favorite foods that you frequently eat. The more you practice, the more control you'll have over your portion sizes when eating to the pyramid.

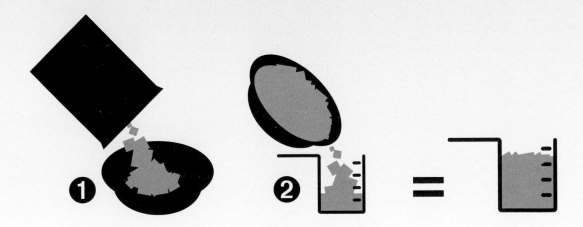

Keeping portions in check

For some people, eating smaller portions (except for vegetables and fruits!) can be a challenge, especially at first. After a while, though, most people get used to their new portion sizes and they find themselves satisfied eating less. Here are a few tips to help you control the portions of food you eat as you adjust to your new normal:

+ **Eat slowly.** When you eat too fast, your brain doesn't get the signal that you're full until it's too late and you've already overeaten.

+ **See what you eat.** Don't eat directly from a container. Seeing food on a plate or in a bowl gives you a better sense of portion size.

+ **Focus on your food.** Watching television, reading or working while you eat distracts you. Before you know it, you've eaten more than you want to. Focus on what you're eating.

+ **Serve smaller amounts.** Take slightly less than what you think you'll eat. Using a smaller plate or bowl makes less food seem like more.

+ **Don't feel obligated to clean your plate.** Stop eating as soon as you feel satisfied. Those extra bites of food that you're trying not to waste add unneeded calories. Better yet, take smaller portions to begin with so you don't waste food.

Chapter 9
Create your eating plan

Go ahead and set aside the food scales and the calculators. *The Mayo Clinic Diet* is designed to help you achieve weight loss with minimal extra gear or equipment. After learning a few key concepts, you're on your way!

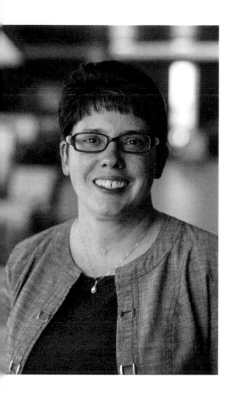

Lisa M. Dierks, RDN
Mayo Clinic
Healthy Living Program

You've done all of the preparation and now it's time to put your plan into action — to start eating to the pyramid and the dining table.

Meal planning is an important ingredient of a successful eating program, but the idea of planning and preparing meals scares many people. They worry it will take too much time, and they're short on time already. They fear it will require significant cooking skills, and cooking is not their forte.

Eating healthy doesn't have to be complicated or time-consuming, but it's important that you follow a few basic rules.

+ Have a general idea of what you'd like to eat during the week ahead so that you have the right foods on hand.

+ Keep your serving targets in mind as you plan your meals. Picture the base of the pyramid — fruits and vegetables. How can you eat more of these each day?

+ Don't forget portion control. Know which foods you can eat more of and which you'll need to limit.

+ Plan ways to use leftovers or healthy, prepackaged foods to build a meal when time is tight.

In the pages that follow, we'll give you helpful tips on meal planning and portion control.

A common theme that comes through loud and clear from people wanting to lose weight is that time is of the essence. "I'm busy. Please don't give me complicated eating plans. I don't have time to measure every ounce or count every calorie."

Eating healthy doesn't have to be complicated. But you'll need to learn which foods to eat and how much of them you can eat so that your meals follow the Mayo Clinic Healthy Weight Pyramid and you have the correct portions on your plate.

To help you with this, you'll learn in this chapter how to plan daily meals and how to estimate portion sizes. There are a number of visual guides in the pages ahead to help train your brain to estimate at a glance how many pyramid servings are on your plate, and in which pyramid food groups they should be counted.

If you can control portion sizes and follow your targeted pyramid servings, you don't need to worry about counting calories because the calories will automatically fall into place.

Eating to the pyramid and dining table

Following the eating recommendations of the Mayo Clinic Healthy Weight Pyramid is actually pretty simple. Turn the page and take a look at the pyramid. Its shape gives you a general idea of what and how much to eat. Focus primarily on the bottom — the vegetables and fruits. These foods are low in energy density (calories per amount of food). That means you can eat a lot of them because they don't contain a lot of calories.

That's why it's recommended you eat more vegetables and fruits than any other food — they provide the least amount of calories per volume. (In Chapters 14 and 15 you'll learn more about energy density, the key principle behind the Mayo Clinic Healthy Weight Pyramid and the Mayo Clinic Healthy Dining Table.)

As you go up the pyramid, the food groups become progressively higher in energy density. To lose weight or manage your weight, you want to eat less of them. That's why whole grains, lean protein and dairy, healthy fats, and sweets have limits as to how much you should consume each day.

So, how does all of this work? First, review the chart on page 86 to determine what your starting calorie target is. Then turn to the chart on page 87 to review how many servings from each of the food groups you should eat each day. Write these numbers down on a piece of paper to keep handy.

For example, if your daily calorie target is 1,200, you can eat unlimited vegetables and fruits, but try to get at least four servings of vegetables and three servings of fruit each day. In addition, you want to eat four carbohydrates servings, three protein and dairy servings and three fat servings.

Unlike with vegetables and fruit, the recommended servings for the other food groups are upper limits — they're not to be exceeded. Granted, no one is perfect and on occasion you're going to slightly exceed them, but the closer you can stick to your target servings, the greater the likelihood you'll achieve your weight goals.

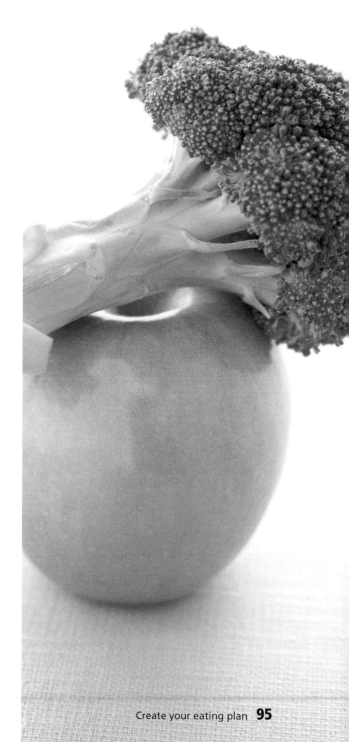

The Healthy Dining Table graphic helps you visualize what your meals should look like on your plate. It shows approximately how your servings should be divided at each meal. For example, at dinner you might have a salad that contains two servings of lettuce or other greens, and on your main plate, two servings of broccoli (a serving of broccoli is ½ cup). That's four servings of vegetables. Your recommended servings are taken care

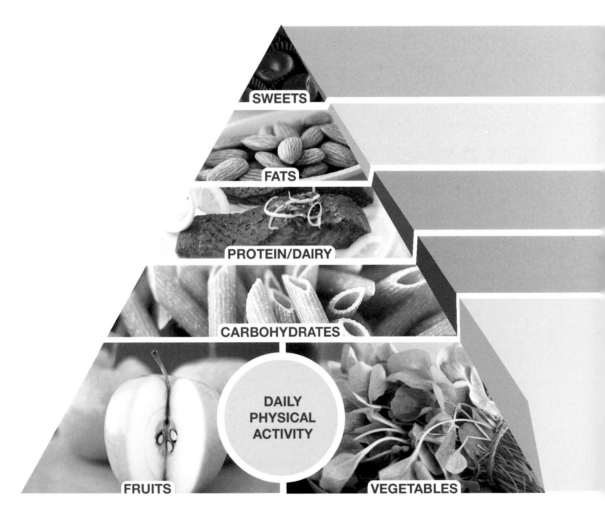

Mayo Clinic Healthy Weight Pyramid

of in one meal! Keep in mind that your table setting will look different for other meals, such as breakfast and lunch, but use the graphic below to create an image in your mind of how much from each food group to eat.

Planning your meals

Now that you know approximately how much, next up is deciding what to eat to meet your servings targets. There are a couple of ways you can do that.

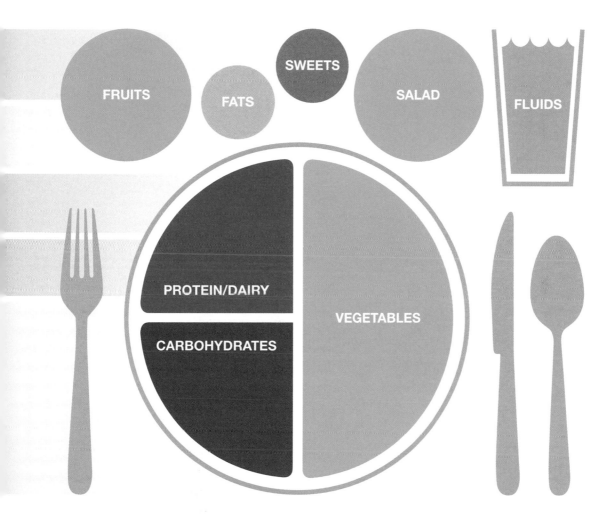

Mayo Clinic Healthy Dining Table

Menu guide

At the back of this book is a section called Menu Guide (see page 300). The Menu Guide contains four weeks' worth of meals — breakfast, lunch, dinner and a snack. You can start at Day 1 and follow the daily menus each day. If you do that, you'll get the right number of recommended servings for all of the food groups.

A note. These menus are designed for individuals aiming to consume approximately 1,200 calories each day. If your daily calorie goal is higher, you'll need to adjust the servings for some of the food groups to hit your daily target.

For instance, if your daily calorie goal is 1,400 calories, you'll need to include one more carbohydrate serving and one more protein/dairy serving, as outlined in the chart on page 87.

On Day 1, that might mean having a whole baked potato for dinner instead of just half a potato and doubling the amount of smoked turkey in your lunch wrap or replacing the calorie-free beverage with a cup of skim milk.

Servings lists

If you would rather have more freedom to choose what you eat, another option is to build your own daily menus. Go to the section at the end of the book called Pyramid Servings (see page 256). It lists a variety of foods in each of the food groups and tells you how much of each equals a serving. Use these lists to plan your menus.

Say for breakfast you have a bowl of cereal, a piece of toast and some fruit. If you look under carbohydrates, you'll see that $3/4$ cup of flake cereal equals one carbohydrate serving. Add 1 cup of skim milk to the cereal and you've added one protein and dairy serving. If you go back to the carbohydrates list you'll see a slice of bread equals another carbohydrate serving. Add in a banana and you have a fruit serving.

With your breakfast you tallied up two carbohydrate servings, one protein and dairy serving and one fruit serving. That means for the rest of the day you have left: two carbohydrate servings, two protein and dairy servings and three fat servings. Plus, you want to eat at least two more fruit servings and at least four vegetable servings. (Remember that the servings goals for vegetables and fruits are minimums, not maximums.)

After you've planned breakfast, plan your lunch and then your dinner, and don't forget to include a snack. When you're done, if you've included too many servings of one food group and not enough of another, go back and tweak things until you get the servings amounts right.

At first, planning your meals may be time-consuming because it's a new process. After a bit, you'll get the hang of it, and you'll become much faster at knowing how to pick and choose foods to reach the right serving amounts.

Combination method

Another option is combining both approaches. Use the Menu Guide for planning your meals, but if one day's menu contains a food item you don't like, swap out that item or meal for something you prefer. You can use the food lists in the Pyramid Servings

Tools to help you

There are a number of tools that can help you plan and track your daily servings. You can use The Mayo Clinic Diet Journal, a soft-cover workbook designed to accompany this book. It provides meal planning tips and pages to record your food servings to make sure you meet your daily goals.

You can also go online and create an account on the Mayo Clinic Diet website (diet.mayoclinic.org) or use The Mayo Clinic Diet mobile app on your phone or tablet.

If none of these appeal to you, a pencil and paper work just as well — maybe a notebook designated especially for this purpose. Or if you find another app or tracker that you like and that works well for you, use that. The important thing is to find the tool that works best for you and fits your needs.

section to help come up with a meal that has the same number of food servings as the one you're replacing.

With time, all of this will become automatic and you won't need to follow the menus or check the food lists as often or at all. You'll know what foods to eat and about how much of each food to keep close to your calorie limit.

Making the process easier

Here are some additional tips to consider as you create your eating plan:

+ **Plan by the week.** It's more efficient to plan menus for an entire week instead of day to day. Don't get hung up on exact servings totals. If you're off target one day, make up for it on the next. Balance things over a week. Use the menu planners in *The Mayo Clinic Diet Journal* to help you plan.

+ **Make pleasure a priority.** Be sure to eat things you like. Losing weight may require you to cut back on some of your favorite foods, but don't sacrifice enjoyment. That

means no severe restrictions, no extreme hunger and no unrealistic expectations. Create some new favorites — there are a lot of great foods and recipes to explore!

+ **Establish a routine.** Let the rhythm of your weekly schedule determine which evenings to spend more time preparing dinner and which evenings to fall back on a convenience food (a healthy one, of course). Save time by using a slow cooker. Make dishes on the weekends and refrigerate or freeze portions for the week ahead.

You might schedule a regular spaghetti night or a leftovers night — based on the extra portions you made at a previous meal. Don't hesitate to repeat the same menus every few weeks.

+ **Adapt menus to the season.** Use the freshest foods available for your meals — asparagus, peas and cherries in the late spring; tomatoes, corn and peaches in late summer. Recently harvested produce is often available at local farmers markets.

- **Don't forget convenience.** On days when there's little time to prepare meals, it's OK to use convenience foods such as a favorite frozen entrée or side dish. Just be selective about what you choose. Read the nutrition labels. Don't choose based on calories alone. Look for items that contain real food (not a lot of processed ingredients) and are low in saturated fat and sodium.

- **Be flexible.** Every food you eat doesn't have to be an excellent source of nutrition. It's OK to eat high-fat, high-calorie foods on occasion. The main point is that most of the time you choose foods that promote good health. They're the ones most likely to help you lose weight.

Portions vs. servings

As you'll recall from previous chapters, servings and portions aren't the same thing. A key to losing weight is understanding the difference between the two. A portion is how much food you put on your plate. A serving is a

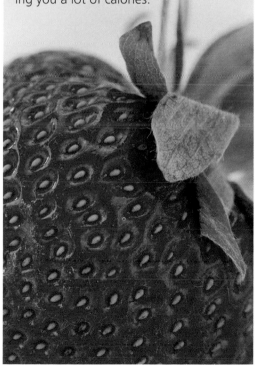

If you're hungry, eat

A cardinal rule of *The Mayo Clinic Diet* is, "If you're hungry, eat!" Starving yourself can be counterproductive and sets you up for overeating later. Plus, it's just no fun.

Because *The Mayo Clinic Diet* allows unlimited consumption of vegetables and fruits, focus on those when you're hungry. They'll fill you up without giving you a lot of calories.

specific amount of food that equals a certain number of calories.

Most people underestimate how many servings are in a portion. They place what they think is a serving on their plate, but it's actually two or more servings. For example, you might consider an 8-ounce steak one serving, but it's actually four servings on *The Mayo Clinic Diet*.

It takes some practice to determine at a glance how many pyramid servings are in a portion. The visuals below are ones you want to memorize because they'll help you select the right amount of food to reach your servings goals. The images in the pages ahead also can help you estimate what equates to a serving.

If this seems like a lot to digest, don't worry. You'll get it! Grab an apple and browse through the next few pages and the sections at the end of the book.

Special diets

If you're on a vegetarian or gluten-free diet, you're in luck. *The Mayo Clinic Diet* is primarily a plant-based diet focused on eating generous amounts of vegetables and fruits, which are naturally gluten-free. And you can still follow the rest of the Healthy Weight Pyramid with just a few small tweaks.

+ **Vegetarian.** If you follow a vegetarian, vegan or other plant-based diet, you might wonder where you'll get your protein servings. If you eat eggs and dairy products, they are good sources, and you don't need to eat large amounts to meet your protein requirements. You can also get sufficient protein from plant-based foods if you eat a variety of them throughout the day. Good plant sources include soy products and

Visual guide to servings sizes
See larger chart on page 89.

1 Vegetable serving =
1 baseball

1 Fruit serving =
1 tennis ball

meat substitutes, legumes, lentils, nuts, seeds, and whole grains.

+ **Gluten-free.** For people following a gluten-free diet, grains that contain gluten, such as wheat, barley and rye, are a primary concern. Yes, *The Mayo Clinic Diet* includes whole grains and whole-grain products within the carbohydrates food group, but it also de-emphasizes many refined grain products, which are often made from wheat.

If you need to avoid gluten, there are many ways to get your carbohydrate servings without eating foods made from wheat, barley or rye. Just emphasize gluten-free whole grains, such as wild or brown rice, quinoa, amaranth, flaxseed and buckwheat.

Other carbohydrate sources that are naturally gluten-free include corn, potatoes and winter squash.

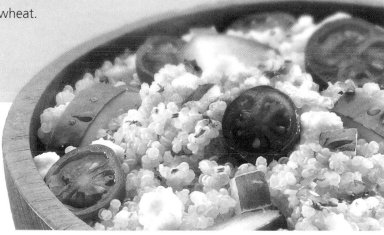

PD Note:
The deck of cards visual cue for the Protein/Dairy group applies only to meat servings. A deck of cards would be too much cheese and too little milk.

1 Carbohydrate serving =
1 hockey puck

1 Protein/Dairy serving =
1 deck of cards or less

1 Fat serving =
1 to 2 dice

Estimating servings

BREAKFAST

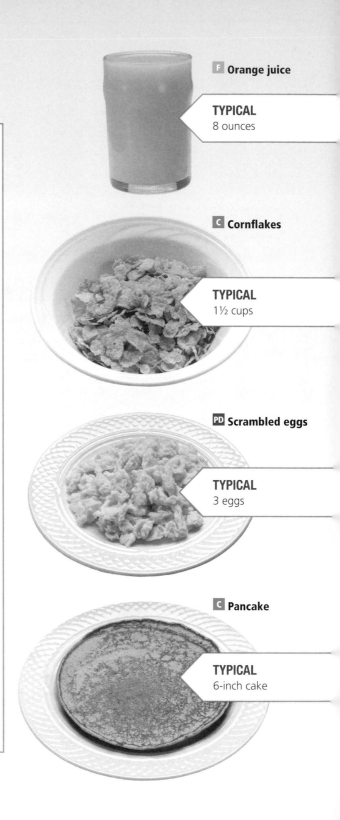

F Orange juice

TYPICAL
8 ounces

C Cornflakes

TYPICAL
1½ cups

PD Scrambled eggs

TYPICAL
3 eggs

C Pancake

TYPICAL
6-inch cake

PRACTICING PORTION CONTROL

Too often, breakfast is an all-or-nothing affair. Either it's calorie overload (eggs, bacon and hash browns) or almost no nutrition at all (coffee or soda). Breakfast should provide you with essential nutrients and give you an energy push. It should not be an occasion for thoughtless or unrestrained eating.

The challenge is to keep your breakfast portions under control. Eating too little deprives you of the important benefits of breakfast. Eating too much simply reduces the number of servings you can eat at later meals in the day.

Typical breakfast portions

Item		Food group	Servings
F	Orange juice	Fruits	2
C	Cornflakes	Carbohydrates	3
PD	Scrambled eggs	Protein/Dairy	3
C	Pancake	Carbohydrates	1½

Tip

Rule to remember!
If you control portion size, the calories tend to take care of themselves.

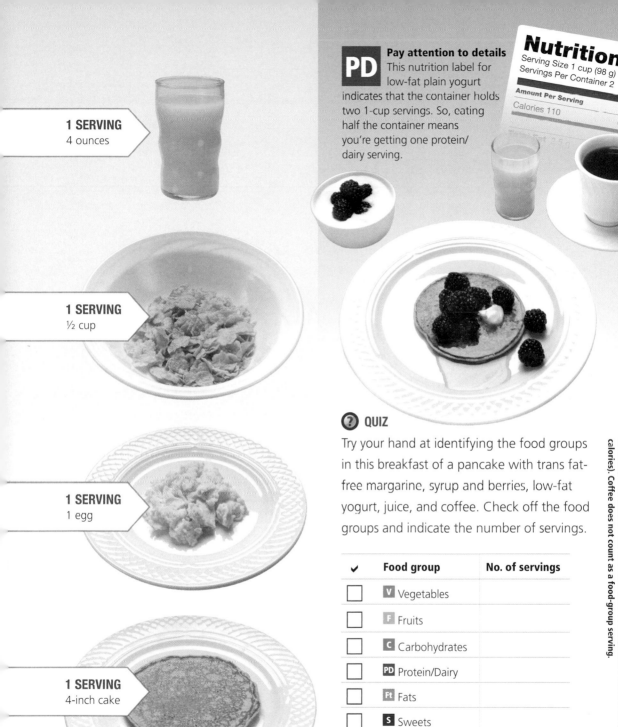

1 SERVING
4 ounces

1 SERVING
½ cup

1 SERVING
1 egg

1 SERVING
4-inch cake

Nutrition Fa
Serving Size 1 cup (98 g)
Servings Per Container 2

Amount Per Serving

Calories 110   Calories fro

? QUIZ

Try your hand at identifying the food groups in this breakfast of a pancake with trans fat-free margarine, syrup and berries, low-fat yogurt, juice, and coffee. Check off the food groups and indicate the number of servings.

✔	Food group	No. of servings
☐	**V** Vegetables	
☐	**F** Fruits	
☐	**C** Carbohydrates	
☐	**PD** Protein/Dairy	
☐	**Ft** Fats	
☐	**S** Sweets	

You'll find the answer on the right-hand side of this page.

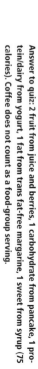

Answer to quiz: 2 fruit from juice and berries, 1 carbohydrate from pancake, 1 protein/dairy from yogurt, 1 fat from trans fat-free margarine, 1 sweet from syrup (75 calories). Coffee does not count as a food-group serving.

Estimating servings

LUNCH

TAKING APART A SANDWICH

If you build something, you can also take it apart, right? One way to estimate servings is to mentally "take apart" the meal. That is, reverse the meal-making process until you can identify the separate ingredients. Try it on something simple, like a roast beef sandwich:

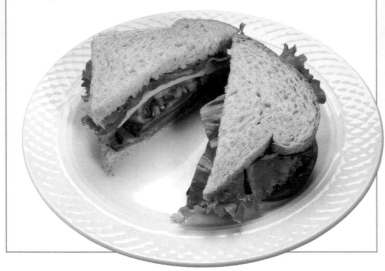

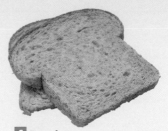

C Bread
1 slice = 1 carbohydrate serving

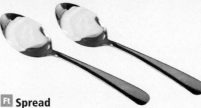

Ft Spread
2 teaspoons of mayonnaise = 1 fat serving

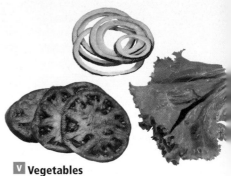

V Vegetables
Tomato slices, onion slice and lettuce = 1 vegetable serving

Here's a breakdown of the food-group servings for your roast beef sandwich:

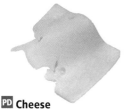

PD Cheese
2 ounces of low-fat cheese = 1 protein/dairy serving

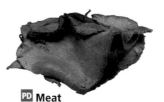

PD Meat
2 ounces of roast beef = 1 protein/dairy serving

V	Vegetables	1
F	Fruits	0
C	Carbohydrates	2
PD	Protein/Dairy	2
Ft	Fats	1
S	Sweets	0

Ft Lose the fat!
Substituting mustard for mayonnaise in your sandwich eliminates the fat serving.

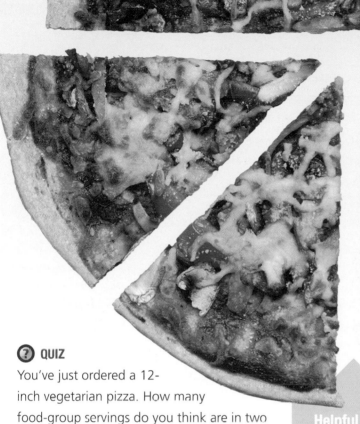

❓ QUIZ

You've just ordered a 12-inch vegetarian pizza. How many food-group servings do you think are in two slices? Put your best guess below:

✔	Food group	No. of servings
☐	**V** Vegetables	
☐	**F** Fruits	
☐	**C** Carbohydrates	
☐	**PD** Protein/Dairy	
☐	**Ft** Fats	
☐	**S** Sweets	

You'll find the answer on the right-hand side of this page.

Helpful hints to deconstruct the pizza:

+ Thin whole-wheat crust
+ Layer of tomato sauce
+ Topped with chopped onion, green pepper and mushroom
+ Sprinkled with low-fat cheese
+ "Hidden" fat used to make the pizza crust

Answer to quiz: 2 vegetables from toppings and tomato sauce, 2 carbohydrates and 2 fats from cheese and pizza crust.

Estimating servings
DINNER

UNSCRAMBLING FOOD JUMBLES

A dish that mixes many ingredients together, such as a stir-fry, can be a special challenge for your food record. It's difficult to know how much of any single food group is a part of the delectable display of colors, shapes, textures and flavors.

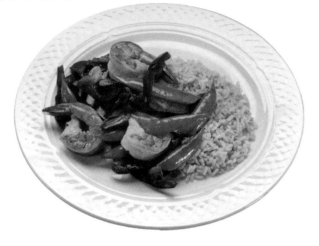

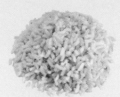

C **Grain**
⅓ cup cooked brown rice =
1 carbohydrate serving

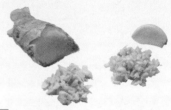

V **Seasonings**
Chopped ginger and garlic =
too little to include as a vegetable serving

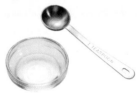

Ft **Oil**
1 teaspoon olive oil = 1 fat serving

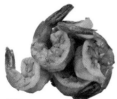

PD **Meat**
4 ounces shrimp
(about 6 large) =
1 protein/dairy serving

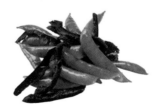

V **Vegetables**
1 medium bell pepper =
1 vegetable serving
¼ cup snow peas =
1 vegetable serving

 In general, about 1 tablespoon of oil is needed for a stir-fry, which equals 3 fat servings. However, most stir-fry recipes serve more than one person.

Here's a breakdown of the food-group servings for the shrimp stir-fry:

V	Vegetables	2
F	Fruits	0
C	Carbohydrates	1
PD	Protein/Dairy	1
Ft	Fats	1
S	Sweets	0

1 Vegetable serving =
1 baseball

1 Carbohydrate serving =
1 hockey puck

1 Protein/Dairy serving =
3 ounces of fish is
1 deck of cards

 QUIZ

How many servings can you estimate for this dinner of grilled salmon, Swiss chard sautéed with olive oil and garlic, and whole-wheat pasta with Parmesan cheese?

✔	Food group	No. of servings
☐	**V** Vegetables	
☐	**F** Fruits	
☐	**C** Carbohydrates	
☐	**PD** Protein/Dairy	
☐	**Ft** Fats	
☐	**S** Sweets	

You'll find the answer on the right-hand side of this page.

Pay attention to your plate

How different foods are served on your dinner plate plays a role in portion control. In general, look for vegetable portions to take up about half the plate and carbohydrate portions about one-quarter of the space. The quarter that remains is for protein/dairy. Add a salad and fruit on the side and you're looking at a pretty healthy meal.

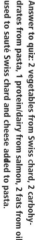

Answer to quiz: 2 vegetables from Swiss chard, 2 carbohydrates from pasta, 1 protein/dairy from salmon, 2 fats from oil used to sauté Swiss chard and cheese added to pasta.

Chapter 10
Expand your
activity plan

If you only cut calories to lose weight — without increasing your physical activity — you lose muscle. Muscle loss makes it harder to keep weight off because muscle tissue burns calories, even at rest. The fastest and most lasting way to lose weight is to alter both parts of the equation — decrease calories in (eating) and increase calories out (physical activity). This chapter will show you how to boost your weight loss by burning more calories.

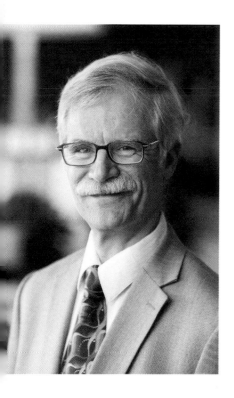

Warren G. Thompson, M.D.
Preventive Medicine

Our ancestors ate more than we do, yet they weighed less. Why? They were always on the move. The television, the automobile, modern appliances and the changing nature of our work — switching from farm labor to desk jobs in front of a computer — have resulted in a dramatic drop in calories burned over the last 100 years.

It is possible to lose weight without being physically active. You may have tried this already — only to regain the pounds you lost, and maybe more. To keep weight off, it's essential that you move more.

Studies have found that people who lose more than 30 pounds and keep it off for five years exercise an hour each day. That may seem like a lot, but it's achievable and it's why our ancestors were thinner. Research also indicates that daily exercise can be hard to maintain. One study of women motivated to lose weight found that two years later only 25 percent were still exercising an hour a day, and they were the only ones who kept their weight off.

Key components of a physical activity program are to:

+ Reduce the time you sit
+ Get more fit
+ Keep at it

The remainder of this chapter will help you implement these key strategies. The changes may seem substantial, but so is the payoff!

Reduce the time you sit

Our ancestors didn't have formal exercise programs. Time spent laboring in fields and factories, or cooking, cleaning and gardening kept them active. Even though they ate more calories than we do today, they weighed less because they sat less.

Compared to just five decades ago, people today move less. At work, where many of us sit at our desks for hours, we're burning an average of 130 fewer calories a day. We're less active at home as well, where it's all too tempting to park ourselves in front of the TV for the evening. And with conveniences like online shopping, banking and socializing, we hardly need to leave the comfort of our chairs.

All that inactivity adds up. On average we spend half our days sitting, and it's taking a toll. Prolonged periods of sitting are associated with an increased risk of health problems such as diabetes, heart disease and some cancers — not to mention weight gain and obesity. Sitting for hours a day

without a break can also be a killer on your spine, leading to low back pain.

And while regular exercise is important to weight loss, unfortunately it doesn't seem to overcome the long-term health effects of too much sitting. As an example, people who sit for eight hours or more a day have an increased risk of heart disease even if they exercise an hour daily.

Moving more at work

You don't need to overhaul your entire workday to move more; you just need to be more proactive. If your job involves a lot of sitting, make a point of breaking up your day by walking around or stretching for a few minutes before you sit back down.

Another strategy is to attach small movements to simple tasks. On the phone a lot? Walk while you're talking. Checking emails often? Stand up when you're reading them or stretch whenever you hit "send."

Changing your office setup can also increase your amount of physical

Adding activity to your day

Take advantage of every opportunity to get up and move around. Here are some simple ways to put more activity into your day. See Chapter 19 for more ways to burn calories.

At home

+ Manually wash your car.
+ Use hand tools instead of power tools.
+ Rake leaves instead of using a blower.
+ Vacuum carpets and dust the furniture.
+ Dance to music when doing chores.
+ Move about while talking on the phone.
+ Go for a short walk before breakfast or walk after dinner.
+ Stretch, walk on a treadmill or use an exercise bike while watching TV.
+ Walk on your treadmill while reading.
+ Go to the mall instead of shop online.

At work

+ Park a few blocks from the office or get off the bus or subway early and walk.
+ Take the stairs, not the elevator, at least for the first few floors — up and down.
+ Walk during your lunch break.
+ Get up and visit your co-workers instead of emailing them.
+ Do stretching exercises or light calisthenics at your desk.

+ Walk around your office while talking on the phone.
+ Use a workstation that combines a treadmill with a computer, so you can walk while working.
+ Spend some of the day at a standing desk or use a stability ball instead of a chair.

Out and about

+ Park a little farther from your destination and walk.
+ Bike or walk to the store.
+ Join a local recreation center.
+ Walk around the field, rink or court while watching a sporting event.

While traveling

+ Take a walk around the terminal while you're waiting for your flight (and don't use the moving walkways!).
+ Do abdominal crunches, pushups and stretching exercises in your hotel room.
+ Get up a little early and walk around the neighborhood or your hotel.

activity. If you trade in your chair for a stability ball, you'll activate your core muscles and use more energy by lightly bouncing. If you have access to a treadmill desk or workstation, try to spend at least part of your day working there.

Moving more at home

At the end of a long day, most of us look forward to some downtime, whether it's watching TV, surfing the internet or playing computer games. Like anything, though, moderation is key. Before seeking out that recliner, do something to get yourself moving. Go for a walk around your neighborhood, clean up the garage or sweep up the house. If you can get the whole family moving with a game of tag or bean bag toss, better yet.

When doing chores around the house or in the garage, put an extra spring in your step by turning on some lively music. And when it's time to enjoy that downtime, consider incorporating some physical activity. Stretch, walk on a treadmill or use a stationary bike for an hour while streaming a movie

or watching TV. Or get up and move during commercials.

Looking for other ways to get moving? Check out the strategies on page 113. Which ones will work for you?

Get more fit

Physical activity is any movement you do that burns calories — whether it's gardening, walking, or stretching during a work break. *Exercise* is a structured, repetitive form of physical activity that improves fitness — such as swimming laps, bicycling, brisk walking and lifting weights.

Any activity that causes you to burn calories is good. You don't have to become an ultimate athlete, but you will benefit by finding creative and enjoyable ways to move more and sit less.

The more active you are, the more calories you'll burn and the more fit you'll become. For example, walking 4 miles in an hour will burn around 350 calories; whereas, running 4 miles in 30 minutes will burn about 500 calories (the exact numbers vary by age, sex, fitness and weight).

But what if you don't like to run or you're not physically capable? You have to consider what's realistic for you given such constraints as your schedule and your health. You'll also need to balance intensity with enjoyment. If you don't enjoy what you're doing, you probably won't keep it up. And keeping it up is key to long-term weight management.

Another pitfall many people fall into is the "terrible toos" — doing too much too fast for their level of fitness. They aren't able to maintain such vigorous exercise, and they soon give up. Remember, you have to walk before you can run!

If you're starting from a relatively low level of fitness, ease into increased activity, allowing your overall fitness to improve over many months. It's better to start slowly and gradually increase your effort and your intensity level. Another reason not to do too much too soon is to avoid injuring yourself.

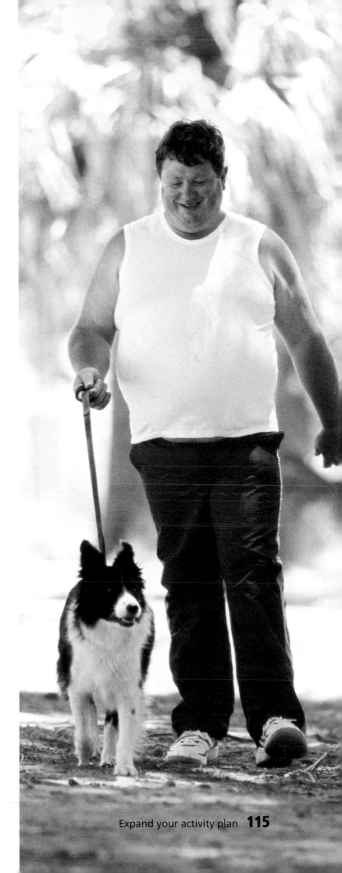

Begin with walking

So, how do you get going? A simple walking program may be your best bet to add more physical activity to your life, especially if you haven't been particularly active. Start out with slow, short walks and gradually increase the frequency, duration and intensity, in that order.

You might begin by walking 30 minutes a day three or four days a week and sitting less at work and home. Gradually increase the number of days you walk until you're walking every day. After a few weeks, when you're feeling more energetic, you may want to walk for 45 minutes some or most days. Or maybe you stay with 30 minutes but try to walk faster. If you're getting a little bored, consider adding another activity to your weekly routine to mix things up. How about a water aerobics class or some bicycling?

Give yourself time to warm up before exercise by starting at a slow pace. Cool down afterward with easy walking or gentle stretching. At least five minutes is recommended for warming up and another five minutes for cooling down.

Break things up if you have to. You don't have to fit all your day's exercise into one session. Three 10-minute exercise sessions a day is almost as beneficial as one 30-minute session.

Keep at it

Gyms and workout facilities often are filled to capacity on January 2. Unfortunately, come February, a lot of people already have dropped out. Starting and sticking to an exercise program can be challenging. Use these tips to help you keep at it!

+ **Do what you love.** If you want an exercise program that you'll stay with, the program should be filled with activities that you enjoy. Many forms of activity can increase your fitness level. The trick is choosing ones that also stimulate and entertain you. Don't train for a marathon if you dislike running!

+ **Pick a time and stick with it.** Schedule specific times to exercise, whether it's for a full afternoon workout or at short, regular intervals. Write the times in your day calendar or journal (in pen, not pencil) **JOT IT** ▸ and remind yourself with notes or a watch alarm. Don't try to fit exercise into your "spare time." If you don't make it a priority, exercise will be pushed aside for other concerns.

+ **Be realistic.** If you aren't a morning person, setting the alarm clock for 4:30 a.m. to get up and exercise before work isn't going to cut it. Don't force yourself into a schedule that doesn't work for you. It won't last.

+ **Find an exercise buddy.** Knowing that someone is waiting for you to show up at the park or the gym is a powerful incentive and can keep you accountable. Working out with a friend, co-worker or family member can bring a new level of motivation to your workouts. Plus, it's nice to have someone to visit with. If you want the motivation of a fitness expert, seek out a personal trainer or exercise classes.

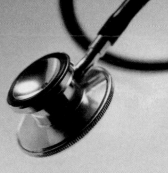

Should you see a doctor?

If you are middle-aged or older, are significantly overweight, or have been inactive for several years, talk to your doctor before increasing your activity level. Your doctor can help you choose activities that are safe and beneficial.

Also consult your doctor before you start exercising if any of the following apply:

+ You have a heart condition and your activity should be medically supervised.
+ You have a family history of heart-related problems before age 55.
+ You have a medical condition requiring a doctor's care.
+ You smoke.
+ You get breathless or experience chest pain after mild exertion.
+ You have frequent dizzy spells.
+ You have severe muscle, ligament or tendon problems.
+ You've been told to reduce your physical activity for any reason.
+ You're taking medications, such as insulin, that may require adjustment if you exercise.

Feeling sore?

Mild muscle soreness following exercise is common, especially if you're trying a new activity. This type of discomfort should disappear in a day or two, and mild activity or stretching may help.

Pain during exercise sends a different signal — it can be a warning sign of impending injury. Most of these injuries result from trying to do too much, too fast. If you feel a sudden, sharp, shooting or irritating ache or pain while exercising, back off from whatever you're doing. The pain should go away in a few days. If it doesn't get better, you might want to see your doctor.

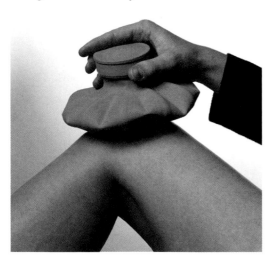

+ **Talk to your family.** You may need your family's help in making time for exercise and to support you on the days you're feeling sluggish. Ideally, it would be best if your family could join you, boosting everyone's health. Plan family outings that include hiking, swimming or skiing.

+ **Gradually increase your exercise.** Studies suggest that to lose weight, you want to aim for at least 300 minutes a week of moderate exercise. That adds up to one hour, five days a week.

+ **Listen to your body.** Exercise shouldn't cause discomfort or pain. If you feel pain, shortness of breath, dizziness or nausea, take a break — you may be pushing yourself too hard. On days that you're generally not feeling well, take a day or two off and resume as soon as you can.

+ **Plan for obstacles.** We all run into obstacles that prevent us from exercising — lack of time, fatigue or boredom. Start by figuring out what your main obstacles are, and then develop some simple strategies to push past them. Having a plan that you can automatically put in place when that obstacle hits is the most successful way to overcome it.

For example, you might realize that surfing the internet after work takes up a lot of your time. Rather than go straight home at the end of the day, head to the gym first or go on a walk. You want to avoid having a debate inside your head about what to do at the end of the day. For more ideas, turn to the Action Guide, beginning on page 234.

+ **Keep track of what you do.** Tracking your physical activity is one of the best ways to keep at it. Studies show that people who monitor their activity are much more likely to stick to an exercise program. In the next chapter, we'll talk about different ways you can track your progress. **JOT IT** ▸

+ **Problem-solve.** Having goals is helpful. If you reach your activity goals, congratulate yourself and move forward. If you didn't reach

your goals, ask yourself why not; don't just give up. If the goals weren't realistic, set goals that are.

For more on exercise and burning calories, see Chapter 19.

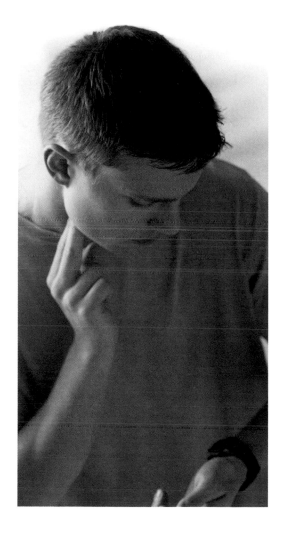

Chapter 11
Track your progress

In these early weeks of *Live It!* you may still be figuring out how to make the *Lose It!* habits part of your everyday life. You're continuing to set goals, make better food choices, and find ways to burn more calories. If you sometimes find it hard to keep track of it all, you're not alone. This chapter will help you get on track!

You may have heard the adage "You can't know where you're going until you know where you've been." Keeping track of your eating and activity routines is important. It helps you identify where you are today so that you can get to where you want to be tomorrow.

Imagine that you're starting a road trip to an amazing location. It would be very helpful to know where the beginning and ending points are, so you can better plan your route. Tracking can help you identify a starting point in your health and fitness journey. Once you know this starting point, you can begin to establish a realistic road map to get to where you want to be in the future.

Many people see tracking as a demonstration of the things that they didn't accomplish. That's not the appropriate mindset. Instead, think of tracking as an opportunity to highlight everything you *did* achieve.

Research has shown that individuals who track their efforts are more successful in reaching their health goals than are those who don't track. It doesn't matter the tool you use to keep records. Tracking can take any shape you desire, and it will help you be mindful of what you're doing to improve your diet and physical activity habits.

Tracking is a valuable tool in your weight-loss toolbox. Use it!

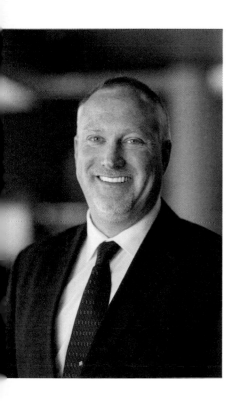

Ryan J. Eastman
Mayo Clinic
Healthy Living Program

These last few weeks you've been working hard to improve your diet and be more active. You may wonder if it's really necessary to write down everything you're eating and doing. The answer is, yes, at least for a while. In this chapter we'll explain why.

Sure, it takes some time and effort, but by tracking your progress you'll gain a lot more than the effort you put in.

Why track?

People tend to significantly underestimate how many calories they consume and overestimate the amount of physical activity they do. Especially in the early stages of your weight-loss plan — when you're still getting a feel for how to eat to the Mayo Clinic Healthy Weight Pyramid — it's easy to misjudge how much you're eating and how active you are.

By keeping accurate food and activity records **JOT IT** ▸, you're more likely to reach your eating and exercise targets and your short- and long-term weight-loss goals. Here are some reasons why tracking is helpful:

+ **Feedback.** Provided you enter information correctly, tracking provides objective feedback on your diet and physical activity efforts, so you can see how well you're sticking with your plan.

+ **Self-awareness.** Tracking makes you more mindful. It helps you to pay attention to what you're putting in your mouth and how much (or little) you're moving your body.

+ **Accountability.** Seeing your eating and activity behaviors in black and white keeps you honest and holds you accountable to yourself.

+ **Reflection.** Tracking is like a mirror. It reveals eating and activity patterns you might not be aware of. Recognizing that unwanted patterns exist is the first step toward overcoming them.

+ **Goal setting.** Having an objective record of where you're at now compared with where you want to be sets you up for success. It allows you to develop small, achievable goals and build on them gradually over time.

+ **Motivation.** When you see that you're meeting your daily and weekly goals and targets, you'll feel inspired to build on those successes.

How to track

There's no wrong or right way to keep food and activity records. What matters is that you choose something that works for you. Most people benefit from a tracking system that's easy to use – not one that's so complicated it becomes an obstacle in and of itself. It should also be something you can keep handy when you need it.

Common tracking tools include:

+ *The Mayo Clinic Diet Journal.*
  The journal is a softcover workbook designed to accompany this book. It provides pages to record what you eat each day, as well as the activities you participate in and for how long. This "low-tech" tool works well for many people.

+ **Apps.** Many smartphone apps allow you to enter the food you eat and measure your physical activity.

Starting at ground zero

If you're reading ahead in this book, know that it's never too early to start tracking your daily eating and physical activity habits. Knowing your baseline patterns — the good and the not so good — can help you set realistic goals as you transition to *Live It!*

Having realistic goals — ones you can actually achieve — will build your confidence and inspire you to stick with your weight-loss efforts.

Use the tips in this chapter for how to keep those records. **JOT IT ▶**

Some apps turn your phone into a pedometer or accelerometer.

+ **Wearable devices.** A wearable fitness tracker can measure what you want to track, such as the number of steps, distance traveled or calories burned. Look for a device that has a long battery life, is waterproof and has a movement alarm that prompts you to move more.

+ **Web-based logs.** The internet offers an abundant source of free or fee-based options for tracking your progress. *The Mayo Clinic Diet* online program is one such option. Whatever you choose, look for a tracking system that allows you to keep food and fitness records in a simple and straightforward way.

+ **Computer-based logs.** For some people simple spreadsheets or word processing documents make the best food and activity logs. Templates for these logs can be found online. Or you can create your own logging system to meet your specific needs.

+ **Paper-based logs.** Many people find that there's no substitute for old-fashioned pen and paper. You can use a basic notebook that's customized to your needs or printouts you find online.

Don't be afraid to experiment. If one tracking system ends up being too cumbersome — or not detailed enough — try another until you find one that's right for you.

Tracking tips

Food and activity records are a great way to monitor if you're meeting your goals and targets discussed in Chapters 7 and 8. To get the most for your efforts:

+ **Experiment.** Don't view your records as do-or-die objectives. Instead, think of them as experiments. You're testing out what works and what doesn't.

+ **Don't fret.** If one day you forget to jot down what you ate or what activities you did, that's OK. Estimate as best you can and get back on track. Just try not to let your forgetfulness become a pattern.

+ **Remind yourself.** If you have trouble remembering to write things down, set up a regular reminder. Maybe it's an email or a chime on your phone or computer that occurs at certain times of the day.

+ **Keep it simple.** Your tracking system doesn't have to be elaborate. All that matters is that you record

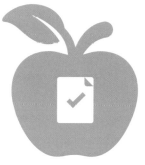

key information that will help you determine if you're meeting your goals and targets.

+ **Do it right away.** You'll be more likely to keep accurate records if you log what you eat right after you eat and exercise. 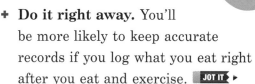 ▶

Start tracking

There isn't a one-size-fits-all formula. It comes down to what works best for you. In the first weeks of *Live It!,* you might find it most useful to log everything you eat and all of your physical activity each day.

Another option, particularly as time goes by, is to track only habits that relate to the targets and goals you're focusing on for the week. So if you feel confident that you're getting enough daily servings of fruits and vegetables but want to cut down on sweets, you might choose to just keep track of the sweets you eat each day. Either way, remember to be honest. The more accurate your records are, the more useful they'll be.

Keep daily food records

People who track what they eat tend to lose more weight. So although keeping daily food records takes some commitment, it's well worth the effort.

Try these tips:

+ **Record amounts.** In addition to what you ate, write down the amount of food you ate, such as a cup of fruit or 4 ounces of salmon. In some cases, you may need to estimate amounts.

+ **Record servings.** Convert the food in your meal into Mayo Clinic Healthy Weight Pyramid food group servings (see pages 256-271). This is how you'll know that you're meeting your daily servings targets. For many of your meals, you may need to break down the entree or side dish into separate food groups (see pages 272-283). A veggie sandwich on whole-wheat bread, for example, might contain two servings from the vegetables group and two from the carbohydrates group.

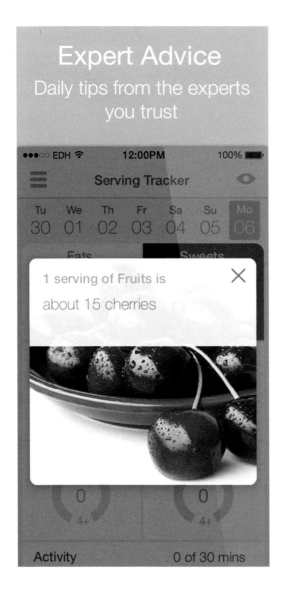

The Mayo Clinic Diet app allows you to track servings and activities, plan your meals and understand portion sizes.

+ **Note the time.** When you record what you eat, also record the time of day. This will help you notice any trends in your eating habits throughout the day.

+ **Don't forget snacks and beverages.** Record everything you put in your mouth, including that handful of chips, a piece of chocolate or a cup of coffee. This also applies to what you munch or sip on while preparing meals.

+ **Include the extras.** Be sure to track ingredients that accompany a food item, such as butter, gravy, ketchup, cheese sauce or salad dressing.

+ **Include other details.** For some people, including additional details is beneficial. If you think it would help you, before eating something record your hunger level on a scale of 1 to 10. You might also make note of your mood — stressed, relaxed, happy or angry. Some people even go so far as to record where they ate the meal and who they ate it with.

This manner of tracking is referred to as a food diary rather than a food record. The additional details can provide you with even broader insights. You might discover that stress is a trigger for eating, that you eat more when you're hanging out at the kitchen counter, or that you always have an afternoon snack, even though you're not that hungry.

Keep daily activity records

Tracking your daily physical activity is equally important. Research shows that people who track their physical activity struggle less with staying physically active, exercise more often and lose significantly more weight. Here are some ways to track how much you're moving **JOT IT** ▸ :

+ **Track all kinds of activity.** Along with structured activities such as walks and aerobic workouts, record other activities that get your body moving. That includes recreational activities such as playing bean bag toss and everyday chores such as cleaning the house, washing the car and weeding the garden.

Calories to servings

There will be times when you may have the calorie information of a food readily available, but it's difficult to deconstruct the item to determine the individual food group servings. In such cases, convert the calories to servings of the food group that the item is closest to.

For instance, if you have a granola bar with a variety of ingredients that's 150 calories, record it has two carbohydrate servings. A carbohydrates serving is 70 calories per serving, so 150 calories would be equivalent to about two servings.

+ **Record the time and distance.** Record how long you do each activity. You can also choose to record the distance you've walked, biked or jogged. For lighter activities, if the activity lasts less than five minutes don't write it down. However, if you're doing something more strenuous, like situps, pushups or walking up flights of stairs, even a few minutes of this type of activity is worth logging in.

+ **Pay attention to intensity.** One way to gauge intensity is to pay attention to how you feel. Notice how hard you're breathing or if your muscles feel fatigued. You can also try measuring your heart rate by checking your pulse or using a heart rate monitor. In general, the higher your heart rate the higher the level of intensity.

+ **Don't go overboard**. When you see blank spaces in your activity record, it's tempting to want to fill them all in. But more isn't necessarily better. If you push yourself too hard, you'll risk injuring yourself or burning yourself out so that you don't want to continue.

+ **Include other details.** If you like writing and don't find the idea intimidating, record one or two good things you experienced during or after the activity or how you could make the activity better.

Record your weight regularly

Weigh yourself regularly and record the results **JOT IT** ▸. How often you step on the scale comes down to personal preference. Some people prefer to weigh themselves daily. Many people prefer to weigh in every few days or once a week. Any of those options can improve your weight-loss efforts as long as you do it consistently.

Don't get caught up in the small ups and downs on the scale. Body fluid levels can fluctuate and change quickly. When this happens, your weight can also change day to day. Such weight fluctuations aren't reflective of real changes in body fat that occur more slowly. Focus on trends over time.

You might also measure and record your waist circumference every few weeks. Your waist size can also tell you whether you're making progress on your weight-loss goals.

Assessing your progress

The beauty of keeping daily records is that you can see where you're going strong and where you can do better. As you examine your records, keep these suggestions in mind:

- **Build on successes.** When you meet a goal, take a moment to celebrate. Then build on that success by modestly increasing your goal.

- **Strategize.** Remember the advice earlier in this chapter to think of new goals as experiments? If you don't meet a weekly goal, instead of getting discouraged, focus on problem-solving. What kept you from reaching the goal? Is it something you can change? Turn to the Action Guide (pages 234-255) for ways to overcome common roadblocks.

- **Look for triggers.** Examine your weekly records for trends you might not be aware of. Are your eating habits worse on the weekends than the rest of the week? Do you snack more during certain times of the day? Being aware of these patterns can help you devise new strategies.

Transitioning from tracking to monitoring

How long you keep food and activity records is up to you. If after a few weeks the task becomes more overwhelming than helpful, it's OK to back off. On the other hand, if keeping daily records continues to motivate you, then stick with it for as long as you like. You might find, for example, that you're ready to pull back on the daily food records after a few weeks but want to keep detailed activity records for several more months, or vice versa.

Your ultimate goal is to develop new, healthier habits so that you can achieve your goals and targets without having to track them.

Once you stop tracking, especially at first, it's still a good idea to monitor how you're doing on a regular basis. You might do this by keeping food and activity records one day a week.

If it appears that you're staying on track, you could reduce that to once every couple of weeks or once a month. This kind of monitoring will help you maintain your self-awareness, hold you accountable and alert you to any new challenges that arise. If you get off balance with a particular goal, you can always go back to recording it more closely until you're back on track.

Chapter 12
Seek support

Studies show that social support is an important part of any lifestyle change, including weight loss. People who have the support of others — friends, family, co-workers, health professionals and individuals trying to make similar lifestyle changes — are more likely to lose weight and to keep it off.

If you're like a lot of people, you may be wary of telling friends, family and co-workers that you're trying to lose weight. In fact, you may be feeling downright shy about the whole thing. That's understandable. The decision to embark on a diet is highly personal and not everyone likes to share personal information.

Perhaps when you were growing up you were teased about your weight, or your personal worth to others seemed to be based on how much you weighed. As an adult, maybe people have questioned your determination, second-guessed your plans to lose weight or even sabotaged your efforts. So, why would you tell people?

Prior negative experiences can be intimidating, but they don't mean that you should go it alone. Research shows you're more likely to be successful if you have the support of others. This chapter offers suggestions on how to build a team of people that can cheer you on, be there for you emotionally, and offer practical strategies and advice to assist you on your way to better health.

Boosting your odds

Receiving support and guidance from others is critical to achieving and maintaining a healthy weight. Too often, people think of being overweight as a personal failure that must be borne and solved alone. But as in so many aspects of our lives, the right type of support can boost our motivation and increase our chances of success.

As you strive to change your lifestyle and improve your weight, there are many ways to receive support and guidance. An honest self-assessment can help determine what's right for you.

Here are some questions to ask yourself as you decide what type of support would be most helpful:

+ Would you prefer a personal coach or being part of a group or class?
+ Are you more motivated when working one-on-one or as part of a larger group?
+ Do group competitions inspire or distress you?
+ Are you more likely to get involved if the setting is in person or virtual?

- Are you more likely to exercise if you do it with a friend or if you enroll in a class?
- Do you have a friend or family member who is looking to make similar lifestyle changes?

Enlisting the help of others can provide many benefits. First, it acknowledges that your intention is worthy of your effort and those whose help you enlist. Second, it gives you a structure to be more accountable to yourself by being accountable to others. Third, it provides a community to encourage you.

The decision to lose weight isn't a one-time decision — it's a daily, sometimes hourly, recommitment. And there will be times when you need some extra strength. In that moment of doubt when an éclair seems like the answer (the co-worker who brings in the donut box every Friday may not be an ally), a quick call to a friend can keep you away from the box.

Plus, having others along can make your journey a lot more enjoyable — and even fun.

Asking for help

Given past negative experiences, asking for help can feel uncomfortable — even frightening. But establishing a network of support can reap powerful rewards. This is especially true when you hit those inevitable bumps in the road.

Research and clinical experiences indicate that people trying to lose weight experience successes, failures, ups, downs and everything in between. Having a team of supporters can help keep you on track during difficult and challenging times.

Some members of your team will be the people closest to you, such as your spouse or best friend. Others might come from unexpected corners of your life — a co-worker who's striving to be more active or a long-distance relative who's also trying to get healthy.

Emotional vs. practical support

As you consider who would be the best people to help you, consider the different types of support you'll need.

Helpful support tends to fall into two categories: emotional and practical. If you've eaten three cookies and want someone to vent to without feeling judged, that's emotional support. If you're looking for someone to walk with you every evening after dinner, that's practical support.

Some people are good at giving both kinds of support, but you'll find that many people in your life are better at one or the other — and that's OK. You're building a team and as with any team, each member has a different role to play.

Building your team

Having a small team to support you provides variety in the type of encouragement you receive, and it prevents one person in your life from being stretched too thin. So how do you go about asking for help from your significant other, family, friends and co-workers? Try these ideas:

+ **Brainstorm.** Make a list of everyone you can think of who might be a source of support. List family

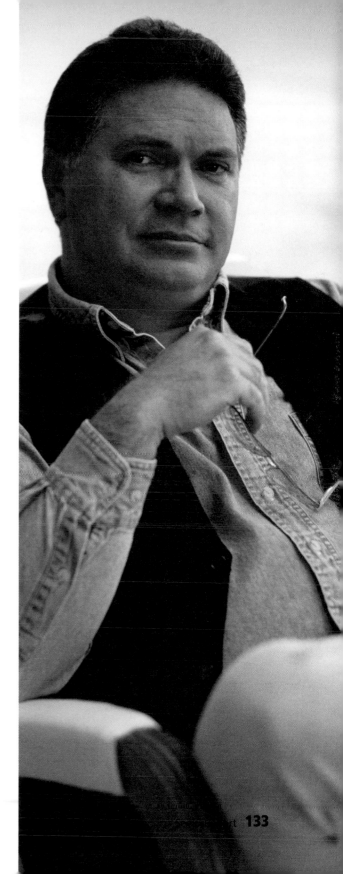

members, friends, co-workers, neighbors and anyone else you have contact with. Don't rule anyone out.

+ **Categorize.** Figure out who's going to be better at offering emotional support and who's more suited to giving you practical support. Your husband might be great when it comes to keeping the kitchen stocked with fruits and vegetables. But your best friend may be a better go-to person when you need a pep talk.

+ **Delegate.** Once you've identified possible supporters, think about specific ways each of them can help you. A dog-owning neighbor might be happy to walk with you every Saturday morning. Your internet-surfing sister might jump at the chance to send you low-calorie recipes she finds online.

+ **Ask.** When you've figured out who you want on your team, reach out to them. Ask them if they would be comfortable supporting you in your weight-loss efforts. Respect their responses.

+ **Show gratitude.** Throughout your weight-loss journey, be sure to thank the people who have committed to helping you. Statements such as, "Thank you so much for listening to me," or "Thank you for walking with me," mean a lot. Most of us don't express thankfulness and gratitude as often as we might.

Getting your family on board

As you strive to lose weight, you may discover that your family is right there with you. They're eating better, too, and coming along on walks and bike rides. This kind of support can be extremely helpful.

But what if those closest to you aren't as supportive? Whether it's a partner who doesn't want to share your lifestyle changes, a mother who insists that you eat her famous dessert or children who resent the sudden lack of treats in the kitchen, knowing how to handle these relationships can help you succeed long term.

Talk to your family. To help gather their support:

How others can help

When friends and family ask what they can do to help, you might not know how to respond. Receiving help may not be something you've dealt with much in the past. Here are some examples of things others can do to help you be successful.

Emotional support	Practical support
Check in weekly to see how you're doing	Keep unhealthy foods out of sight or out of the house
Be a nonjudgmental shoulder to lean on when you've had a bad day	Help out with shopping, meal preparation and cooking
Provide positive feedback and encouragement	Encourage you to eat fruits, vegetables and other healthy foods
Be willing to chat whenever you need a distraction or just want to talk	Be a dependable partner for walks, workouts or other activities you both enjoy

Provide reassurance. It's not uncommon for a partner or companion to feel threatened as you lose weight and improve your appearance. Remind your loved one that while you may be changing your lifestyle, your feelings for him or her haven't changed.

Express yourself. Just as it's good to acknowledge what your loved ones are going through, it's important to let them know how they may be affecting you. Let them know what's helpful and what's not. Discuss how they can best support you.

Seek compromise. Your family may be feeling overwhelmed by all the changes you're making at home, especially if they're directly affected. You're now cooking different foods, bringing different foods into the house and going to exercise classes. These are all changes for them. Look for points of compromise so that you can meet each other halfway. Rather than rid the house of all snack foods, maybe you can agree to avoid the treats that tempt you the most, or ask family members to keep their snacks out of sight.

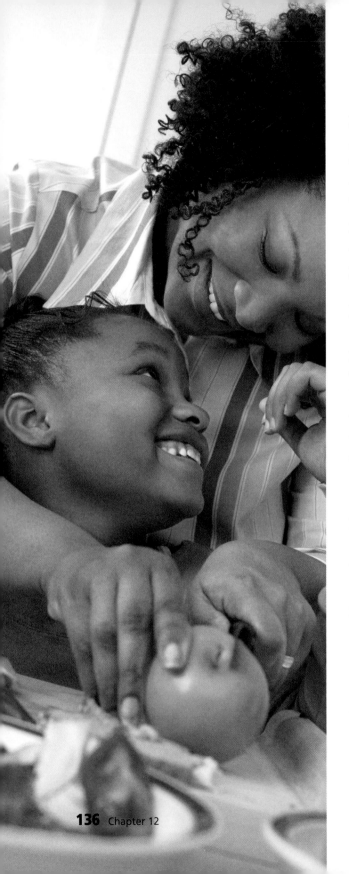

Find the fun. Make a list of recreational activities that you all enjoy and would like to do together. Then schedule time to do them. Everyone will benefit from being active and having more bonding time. Going to the beach or on walks, hikes or bike rides are just a few examples.

Keep the conversation going. Continue to talk about any concerns you have and give your family a chance to do the same. Keep an open mind. Be willing to problem-solve together when difficulties or frustrations come up. As stated earlier, express thankfulness and gratitude when family members do support you.

Reach out. If you're struggling with specific family dynamics, call on your weight-loss partners or seek out a support group. These people can help you counteract the temptations or negative messages you're receiving.

Other types of support

When it comes to weight loss, there are four main sources of support. Each has a critical role to play:

- Your spouse or significant other
- Your family and friends
- A health care provider
- A support group

We've talked about enlisting the help of your significant other and family members and friends. Equally important are two other types of support — the type you get from a health care provider and the type provided by support groups. Extending your support network to include these two areas increases your odds of success.

Provider support

Having a health care provider in your court is a great asset. Think about whom you'd be most comfortable turning to for questions or concerns throughout your weight-loss journey and who has helped you in the past. It might be your primary care doctor, a nurse practitioner, a psychologist, a dietitian, or someone else you see on a regular or occasional basis.

Even if you only see this person once a year, support from a health care provider can be tremendously helpful.

Knowing you have a source of expert advice can boost your confidence and help you stay on track with your weight-loss plan.

This person can also keep you informed about other positive changes to your health. Being told that your cholesterol level has dropped by 20 points can be very motivating!

Support groups

It can be tremendously helpful to share stories and ideas with others who are on the same journey — people who are trying to change their behaviors and lose weight just like you are. There's nothing like talking to someone who knows exactly what you're going through.

A support group can be a vital part of your support network. But it's important that it be the right type of group. There are a lot of support groups and chat rooms available online. Some of these groups may not provide the best information, or they might be trying to promote a program that's not safe or right for you.

Finding a fitness buddy

One of the best ways to stay motivated and meet your weight-loss goals is to team up with a dependable fitness partner. Knowing that another person is counting on you to show up for an activity can kick you into gear when you're feeling sluggish and unmotivated. A fitness buddy can also talk with you while you're exercising — and make the experience more enjoyable. Consider these factors when thinking about who might be a good fitness buddy for you:

Commitment. Look for someone who's motivated to keep active. You want a partner who will nudge you when you're stuck on the couch, and who counts on you to do the same for him or her.

Goals. You should have similar goals and interests. This will help when deciding the types of physical activities to do and the amount of time you spend doing them.

Companionship. This person will be someone you'll spend a lot of time with. Your fitness buddy doesn't have to be your best friend — or even a close friend or family member. It just has to be someone you enjoy spending time with.

Comfort. Your fitness buddy should make you feel at ease, not insecure. It's OK if you're not at the exact same fitness level. In fact, exercising with someone a little more fit than you can be motivating. But if you think you'll be comparing yourself to this person in a negative way, he or she probably isn't the right match for you.

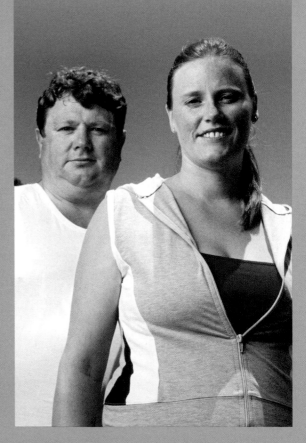

Look for a group that's led by a health care professional — a person who can offer sound medical advice — and for a group that meets regularly from week to week. How do you find such a group? Try these options:

+ **Ask your doctor.** He or she might know of a weight-loss group that meets at a local clinic or community center.

+ **Call your community hospital.** Many hospitals offer regular meetings and informational sessions for people trying to lose weight.

+ **Check at your workplace.** Some workplaces sponsor weight management groups that are professionally led. Yours might be one of them.

+ **Inquire at the gym.** Some fitness centers offer weekly health and nutrition classes to members.

If it's not possible to take part in a professional group, you might consider forming a virtual support group. Such a group might include a small number of co-workers all trying to manage their weight. The group may create an email distribution list that everyone can participate in to answer questions, share ideas and recipes, and respond to a member who's having a bad day.

Be your No. 1 supporter

While you're busy creating and maintaining a support network, it's easy to forget about your most important supporter — that's you. Believe in yourself and treat yourself with the same compassion and kindness you seek from others.

Don't beat yourself up on days when things don't go well. Everyone has a bad day now and then. The key is to learn from those mistakes without dwelling on them. Remind yourself that you're only human, that you can learn from your mistakes and that you'll do better tomorrow.

It's also important to stay positive. If you find yourself trapped in negative thoughts, replace them with positive ones. Turn the message that says, "I'll never succeed at this" into one that says, "I'm not giving up."

Part 3
All the Extra Stuff

Lose It! and *Live It!* are the *doing* parts of *The Mayo Clinic Diet.* Part 3 gives you important support information.

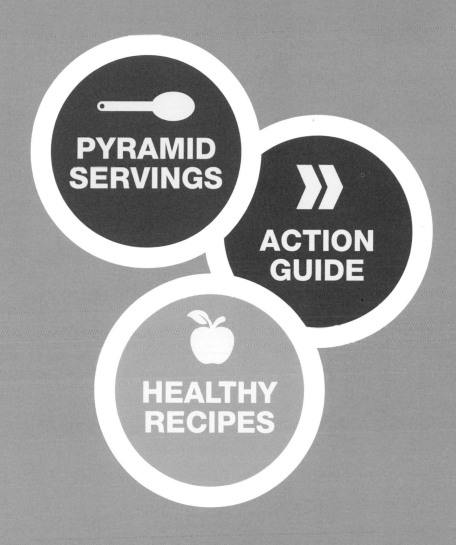

PYRAMID SERVINGS

ACTION GUIDE

HEALTHY RECIPES

Chapter 13
What's your healthy weight?

How much *should* you weigh? Well, that's not an easy question, and there's no one-size-fits-all answer. The right weight for you is unique to you and dependent on a number of factors (including — but not solely — what you *want* to weigh). And, of course, your health is an important part of the equation. This chapter will help you weigh the considerations.

You probably already know why you *want* to lose weight, but do you *need* to lose weight?

"Hey, just look at me! Isn't it obvious?" may be your answer.

Maybe. Maybe not.

Looks certainly play a role in determining the right weight for you. How you look helps shape your self-image, and that can affect your mental health. Looks are a valid consideration — as long as you're keeping things in proper perspective.

But for a moment, put aside how you look in a mirror (or a swimsuit) and consider another critical factor — your overall health.

Being at a weight that's good for your health — what we'll call a *healthy weight* — can reduce your risk of a variety of diseases, help you live longer and improve the way you feel. And oh, it may just improve the way you feel about how you look.

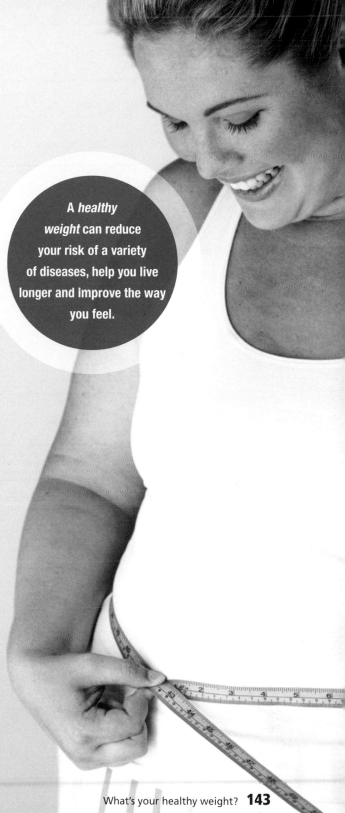

A *healthy weight* can reduce your risk of a variety of diseases, help you live longer and improve the way you feel.

What is a healthy weight?

Simply put, a healthy weight means you have the right amount of body fat in relation to your overall body mass. It's a weight that allows you to feel energetic, reduces your health risks, helps prevent premature aging (such as worn-out joints from carrying around too much weight) and improves your quality of life.

Stepping on the scale only tells you your total weight — including bone, muscle and fluid — not how much of your weight is fat. The scale also doesn't tell you where you're carrying that fat. In determining health risks, both of these factors are more important than is weight alone.

So how do you know if you're at a healthy weight? While there are no objective standards for what weight "looks good," there are standards for what determines a healthy weight.

The most accurate way to determine how much fat you're carrying is to have a body fat analysis. This requires a professional using a reliable method of estimation, such as weighing a person underwater or using an X-ray procedure called dual energy X-ray absorptiometry. Either method can be expensive and fairly complicated. A procedure called bioelectric impedance analysis is more widely available, but its accuracy can vary.

The most common method to determine if your weight is healthy is by using the National Institutes of Health threefold approach:

+ Your body mass index (BMI)
+ The circumference of your waist
+ Your personal medical history

Body mass index (BMI)

BMI is a tool for indicating your weight status (see the opposite page). The mathematical calculation takes into account both your weight and height. Although BMI doesn't distinguish between fat and muscle, it more closely reflects measures of body fat than does total body weight.

Although a BMI number tends to correlate with body fat for most people,

What's your BMI?

To determine your BMI, find your height in the left column. Follow that row across to the weight nearest yours. Look at the top of that column for your approximate BMI. Or use this formula:

1. Multiply your height (in inches) by your height (in inches).
2. Divide your weight (in pounds) by the results of the first step.
3. Multiply that answer by 703. (For example, a 270-pound person, 68 inches tall, has a BMI of 41.)

	Normal		Overweight					Obese				
BMI	**19**	**24**	**25**	**26**	**27**	**28**	**29**	**30**	**35**	**40**	**45**	**50**
Height							Weight in pounds					
4'10"	91	115	119	124	129	134	138	143	167	191	215	239
4'11"	94	119	124	128	133	138	143	148	173	198	222	247
5'0"	97	123	128	133	138	143	148	153	179	204	230	255
5'1"	100	127	132	137	143	148	153	158	185	211	238	264
5'2"	104	131	136	142	147	153	158	164	191	218	246	273
5'3"	107	135	141	146	152	158	163	169	197	225	254	282
5'4"	110	140	145	151	157	163	169	174	204	232	262	291
5'5"	114	144	150	156	162	168	174	180	210	240	270	300
5'6"	118	148	155	161	167	173	179	186	216	247	278	309
5'7"	121	153	159	166	172	178	185	191	223	255	287	319
5'8"	125	158	164	171	177	184	190	197	230	262	295	328
5'9"	128	162	169	176	182	189	196	203	236	270	304	338
5'10"	132	167	174	181	188	195	202	209	243	278	313	348
5'11"	136	172	179	186	193	200	208	215	250	286	322	358
6'0"	140	177	184	191	199	206	213	221	258	294	331	368
6'1"	144	182	189	197	204	212	219	227	265	302	340	378
6'2"	148	186	194	202	210	218	225	233	272	311	350	389
6'3"	152	192	200	208	216	224	232	240	279	319	359	399
6'4"	156	197	205	213	221	230	238	246	287	328	369	410

Based on *Circulation*, 2014;129(suppl 2):S102; NHBLI Obesity Expert Panel, 2013.
*Asians with a BMI of 23 or higher may have an increased risk of health problems.

it's not always a good match. Some people may have a high BMI but relatively little body fat. For example, an athlete may be 6 feet 3 inches tall and weigh 230 pounds, giving him a BMI of 29 — well above the classification of healthy weight. But he's not overweight because training has turned most of his weight into lean muscle mass.

By the same token, there may be some people who have a BMI in the "healthy" range but who carry a high percentage of body fat. For most people, though, BMI provides a fairly accurate approximation of health risk as it relates to their weight.

Waist measurement

Many conditions associated with excess weight, such as high blood pressure, abnormal levels of blood fats, coronary artery disease, stroke, diabetes and certain types of cancer, are influenced by the location of body fat.

Fat distribution can be described as apple-shaped or pear-shaped. If you carry most of your fat around your waist or upper body, you're referred to as apple-shaped. If most of your fat is around your hips and thighs or lower body, you're pear-shaped.

In general, when it comes to your health, it's better to have a pear shape than an apple shape. If you have an apple shape, you carry fat in and around your abdominal organs. Fat in and around your abdomen increases your risk of developing disease. If you have a pear shape, your risks aren't as high.

To determine whether you're carrying too much weight around your middle, measure your waist. Find the highest point on each hipbone and measure horizontally around your body just above those points. A measurement exceeding 40 inches in men or 35 inches in women indicates an apple shape and increased health risks.

The table on the opposite page can help you determine whether to be concerned about your waistline.

Although these cutoffs of 40 and 35 inches are useful guides, there's

Is your health at risk?

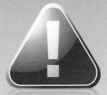

If your BMI is less than 18.5, talk with your doctor. You may be at risk of health conditions associated with a low body weight. A BMI of 18.5 to 24.9 is considered a healthy range, however Asians with a BMI of 23 or more may have an increased risk of health problems. If your BMI is 25 or higher, see the table below.

Weight-related risk of disease

IF	Your body mass index (BMI) is ▾	&	Your waist measurement is ▾	
			Women: 35 inches or less Men: 40 inches or less	Women: Over 35 inches Men: Over 40 inches
Overweight	25-29.9		Increased risk	High risk
Obese	30-34.9		High risk	Very high risk
	35-39.9		Very high risk	Very high risk
Extreme obesity	40 or over		Extremely high risk	Extremely high risk

Source: 2013 AHA/ACC/TOS guideline for the management of overweight and obesity in adults: A report of the American College of Cardiology/American Heart Association Task Force on Practice Guidelines and The Obesity Society; *Circulation*, 2014;129(suppl 2):S102.

nothing magic about them. It's enough to know that the bigger the waistline, the greater your health risks.

Medical history

Your BMI and waist measurement numbers don't give you the full picture of your weight status. A complete evaluation of your medical history also is important. In talking with your doctor about your weight, consider:

+ **Do you have a family history of obesity, cardiovascular disease, diabetes, high blood pressure or sleep apnea?** This may mean increased risk for you.

+ **Have you gained considerable weight since high school?** Even people with normal BMIs may be at increased risk of weight-related conditions if they've gained more than 10 pounds since young adulthood.

+ **Do you have a health condition, such as high blood pressure or type 2 diabetes, that would improve if you lost weight?**

+ **Do you smoke cigarettes or engage in little physical activity?** These factors can compound the risk represented by excess weight.

BMI and waist measurement are snapshots of your current weight. The medical history helps reveal your risk of being overweight or of developing weight-related diseases.

So what's your healthy weight?

If your BMI shows that you're not overweight, if you're not carrying too much weight around your abdomen and if you answered no to all of the medical history questions, there's probably little health advantage to changing your weight. (But you may still improve your health through a healthy diet and physical activity.)

If your BMI is between 25 and 30 or your waist measurement exceeds healthy guidelines, and you answered yes to one or more of the medical history questions, you'll probably benefit from losing a few pounds. Talk to your doctor before you start to lose weight. And if your BMI is 30 or more, you're considered obese. Losing weight should improve your health and reduce your risk of weight-related illnesses.

Now if your analysis shows that you're at a healthy weight, but you're still dissatisfied with the way you look, then you've got some thinking to do. If you're at the middle or upper end of a healthy BMI, there's probably little risk to losing a few pounds. But if you're at the lower end of a healthy BMI range, and losing weight would push you into the underweight category (less than 18.5), then losing weight may put your health at risk.

Why am I overweight?

The simple answer to why anyone is overweight is that they're consuming more calories than they're burning through physical activity. It's a basic mathematical equation in which a number of factors can play a role.

+ **Lifestyle factors.** Eating high-calorie foods, eating large portions, working sedentary jobs, not exercising and use of labor-saving devices can all pack on the pounds.

+ **Genetic factors.** Evidence suggests that obesity runs in some families, but the role genes play is unclear. Scientists believe that obesity is more likely the result of a complex interaction between genes and environment. This means that although you may have a genetic predisposition to being overweight, it's not fate. Ultimately, your weight is determined by the influence of physical and social factors.

+ **Psychological factors.** People sometimes overeat to cope with problems or to deal with emotions such as boredom, sadness and frustration. In some people, a psychiatric illness called binge-eating disorder can contribute to obesity.

+ **Other factors.** These factors may contribute to weight gain but they generally aren't enough in and of themselves to lead to obesity:

▸ **Age** — With age, the amount of muscle in your body tends to decrease, lowering your metabolism. In addition, people tend to be less active as they get older. Both result in fewer calories burned.

▸ **Stopping smoking** — Many smokers gain some weight after stopping smoking, but the benefits of stopping smoking outweigh whatever health risks may result from the weight gain.

▸ **Pregnancy** — Some women gain more weight than recommended during a pregnancy and they may retain it afterward.

▸ **Medication and illness** — Corticosteroids, tricyclic antidepressants, anticonvulsants, insulin and hormones may cause weight gain. Sometimes, alternative medications can be prescribed. Rarely obesity can be traced to an endocrine disorder, such as low thyroid function or Cushing's syndrome. Some medical conditions can interfere with exercise, making weight gain more likely.

Chapter 14
Energy, calories and weight

Carbohydrates, fats, proteins . . . oh my! Sounds like a lot to keep track of. But more than anything, at its core, weight is about *energy* — and the balance between what you take in when you eat and what you burn through physical activity. This chapter gives some depth to that relationship.

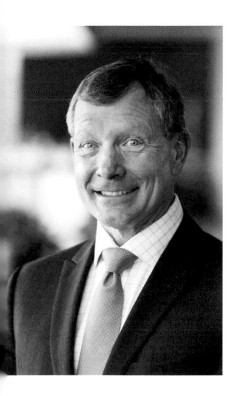

Michael D. Jensen, M.D.
Endocrinology

Most women burn 1,700 to 2,200 calories a day, and most men somewhere between 2,000 and 2,600 calories. Unless you're very inactive or unusually active, you probably fall within these bounds.

Of your daily calories burned, about 30 to 60 percent are from fat. Why is this important? Think of fat calories burned as fat dollars spent from your body's fat bank account. A woman weighing 220 pounds has approximately half a million dollars in her fat bank account. (A pound of fat is equal to 3,500 calories, or fat dollars.) Almost everyone, including this woman, spends less than a dollar a minute from their fat bank accounts. Because men burn calories a bit faster, they tend to have somewhat smaller fat bank accounts.

The main message here is that fat doesn't come off quickly. At the rate most humans burn calories, it's not possible to quickly reduce the size of their fat bank accounts. This doesn't mean, however, that the task is impossible or that you shouldn't try. It just means that losing fat takes time.

You can pretty accurately estimate how many calories you spend a day with an activity monitor, such as a step counter. That will give you an idea of your spending rate. If you reduce the deposits to your fat bank account by eating healthier and consuming fewer calories, or you increase the calories you burn with increased activity, you'll eventually reduce your body's fat bank account to a level you're more satisfied with.

All living things need energy to grow and develop, to function properly, and, in short, to survive. Your body has a constant demand for energy. You replenish energy with the food you eat.

Weight is all about the balance between energy added through diet and energy burned through activity. This energy equation is a basic principle of weight control.

Food energy is measured in units called calories. It's easy to find lists of foods and the calories they contain. Energy burned in activity is also measured in calories, and there are lists to show you how many calories you can burn by doing certain activities. This knowledge is helpful in assessing your energy balance as you try to achieve or maintain a healthy weight.

Tracking calories in and calories out in a journal is helpful in weight loss. **JOT IT** ▸ At first, this may seem like a lot of work, but it's not necessarily something you have to do forever. With practice, you can get to the point where you have a pretty good idea of your energy flow without tracking it.

Dietary sources of energy

The food you eat supplies many types of macronutrients, which provide the energy your body needs to function. These macronutrients include carbohydrates, fats and proteins. Other nutrients, such as vitamins and minerals, don't provide calories but help the body with chemical reactions. Food is also a source of water, fiber and other essential substances.

Carbohydrates

Carbohydrates can be simple or complex. Simple carbohydrates are the sugars found in fruits, honey, milk and milk products. They also include sugars added during food processing and refining. Simple carbohydrates are absorbed quickly for energy.

Complex carbohydrates, also known as starches, are found primarily in whole grains, pasta, potatoes, beans and vegetables. Digestion is required to change complex carbohydrates into simple sugars. Complex carbohydrates contain many vitamins and minerals as well as fiber.

During processing, complex carbohydrates may be refined, removing many important nutrients and their benefits.

Fats

Fats are a natural component of various foods that come in different forms. The oils used in cooking are forms of fat. Fats are also found in foods of animal origin, such as meat, dairy, poultry and fish, and in foods such as avocados, nuts and olives.

Fats are a major source of energy (calories). When your body digests and absorbs fats, it also absorbs some types of vitamins.

Proteins

Proteins build and repair body structures, produce body chemicals, carry nutrients to your cells and help regulate body processes. Excess proteins also provide calories. Proteins are composed of basic elements called amino acids. There are two types of amino acids: those your body can generate (nonessential) and those only obtained from the food you eat (essential).

What's a calorie?

Calories can be used to measure any kind of energy, but people most often associate the term with nutrition. One calorie is the amount of energy required to raise the temperature of 1 gram of water by 1 degree Celsius (1.8 F).

Because that's such a small unit of measure, food energy is measured in kilocalories (1,000 calories). The numbers you see on nutrition labels are still marked as calories because in nutrition, calorie and kilocalorie have become synonymous.

Vitamins

Many foods contain vitamins, such as A, B complex, C, D, E and K. Vitamins help your body use carbohydrates, fats and proteins. They also help produce blood cells, hormones, genetic material and chemicals for the nervous system.

During processing, foods can lose nutrients. Manufacturers may enrich (fortify) products to add back lost nutrients. Natural foods that contain vitamins in their natural state are generally preferred to fortified foods.

Minerals

Minerals such as calcium, magnesium and phosphorus are important to the health of your bones and teeth. Sodium, potassium and chloride, commonly referred to as electrolytes, help regulate the water and chemical balance in your body. Your body needs smaller amounts of minerals such as iron, iodine, zinc, copper, fluoride, selenium and manganese, commonly referred to as trace minerals.

Water

It's easy to take water for granted, but it's a vital nutritional requirement. Many foods, especially fruits, contain a lot of water. Water plays a role in nearly every major body function. It regulates body temperature, carries nutrients and oxygen to cells via the bloodstream, and helps carry away waste. Water also helps cushion joints and protects organs and tissues.

Fiber

Fiber is the part of plant foods that your body doesn't absorb. The two main types of fiber are soluble and insoluble, and fiber-rich foods usually contain both.

Foods high in soluble fiber include citrus fruits, apples, pears, plums and prunes, legumes (dried beans and peas), oatmeal and oat bran, and barley. Soluble fiber helps lower blood cholesterol, slows the rise in blood sugar and adds bulk to stools.

Insoluble fiber is found in many vegetables, wheat bran, and whole-grain breads, pasta and cereals. Insoluble fiber also adds bulk to stool, stimulates the gastrointestinal tract and helps prevent constipation.

Where the calories come from

Carbohydrates, fats and proteins are the types of nutrients that contain calories, and that means they're the main energy sources for your body. The amount of energy each nutrient provides varies.

+ Carbohydrates are the food nutrients that your body uses first. During digestion, they're released into your bloodstream and converted into blood sugar (glucose). When there's a demand, the glucose is absorbed immediately into your body's cells to provide energy.

If there's no immediate demand, glucose can be stored in your liver and muscles. When these storage sites become full, excess glucose is converted into fatty acids and stored in fat tissue for later use.

+ Fats are extremely concentrated forms of energy, and they pack the most calories per ounce. When digested, they're broken down into fatty acids, which are the parts of fat used for energy or for other body processes.

If there's an excess of fatty acids, a small quantity can be stored in your liver and muscles, but most of the excess is stored in fat tissue. The amount of fat that can be stored in fat tissue is usually much greater than can be stored in other tissues.

+ Proteins have many responsibilities, including supplying energy for

Food sources of energy

Fats supply more calories per gram than do carbohydrates and proteins combined. Many people are surprised that alcohol can be such a high source of calories.

Nutrient	Calories (per gram)
Fats	9
Alcohol	7
Carbohydrates	4
Proteins	4

physical activity. This can happen if you consume too few calories, if you eat excess protein, or if you're involved in prolonged physical activity. Any excess calories from protein are converted into fat and stored.

Vitamins, minerals, water and fiber don't contain calories. However, they're still vital to your health and well-being. When they're lacking from your diet, you increase your risk of serious illness.

Your energy account

The energy needs of your body can be viewed like a bank account. Lots of transactions take place. You have daily deposits and daily withdrawals.

Your deposits are food, with three nutrients providing the bulk of your energy: carbohydrates, fats and proteins. When you eat, you're adding calories to your energy account.

Withdrawals can be made in three ways, each of which burns calories:

+ **BMR.** Even when you're in a state of complete rest, your body is using energy to meet its basic needs, such as breathing, blood circulation, and cellular growth and repair. This energy use at rest is called your basal metabolic rate (BMR). Your BMR is responsible for the greatest demand on your energy account — generally, one-half to two-thirds of your total energy expenditure.

+ **Thermic effect of food.** The energy your body uses to digest, absorb, transport and store the food you eat is known as the thermic effect of food. It takes about 10 percent of your total energy use.

+ **Physical activity.** Daily tasks such as getting dressed, brushing your teeth and other routine activities also require energy. At least 30 to 35 percent of your calorie needs should go toward these activities.

The energy use required for BMR and digestion remain relatively steady and aren't easy to change. The best way to increase your energy withdrawal — in other words, to burn more calories — is to increase the amount of physical activity you take part in.

Influences on your energy account

If everyone were physically and functionally identical, it would be easy to determine the standard energy needs for all kinds of activity. But other factors affect your energy account.

Some of the factors that influence your BMR and your overall energy needs are age, body size and composition, and sex.

+ **Age.** Children and adolescents, who are in the process of developing their bones, muscles and tissues, need more calories per pound than do adults. In fact, infants need the most calories per pound of any age group because of their rapid growth and development.

Not surprisingly, as hormone levels and body composition change with age, so does your BMR. By the time you reach early middle age, your BMR and energy needs start declining, generally at a rate of 1 to 2 percent a decade.

+ **Body size and composition.** A bigger body mass requires more energy, and thus more calories, than does a smaller body mass. In addition, muscle burns more calories than does fat, so the more muscle you have in relation to fat, the higher your BMR.

Based on this principle, you can slightly increase your BMR and the amount of energy you burn by building up your muscle mass through regular physical activity.

Empty calories

Empty calories is a term applied to sugar and alcohol. They contribute calories but few other essential nutrients.

Small amounts of alcohol — up to two drinks a day for men age 65 and younger and one drink for all women and for men older than age 65 — have been linked with a lower risk of heart disease.

But excessive drinking can add unwanted pounds, raise blood pressure, damage your liver and increase the risk of some cancers.

One drink equals:

+ One 12-ounce regular beer (150 calories)

+ One 5-ounce glass of wine (about 100 calories)

+ One 1½-ounce shot of 80-proof liquor (about 100 calories — mixes can add more)

+ **Sex.** Men usually have less body fat and more muscle than do women of the same age and weight. This is why men generally have a higher BMR and higher energy requirements than women do.

Balancing your account

Your body weight is a physical reflection of your energy account. Daily fluctuations in weight indicate the daily changes in your account.

If you withdraw from the account approximately the same amount of energy as you deposit, your weight stays the same. If you spend more from the account than you deposit, you lose weight.

There's a magic number in this energy equation. Remember 3,500 calories equals about 1 pound of body fat. To gain a pound you need to consume 3,500 more calories than you burn, and to lose a pound you need to burn 3,500 calories more than you consume.

The tricky part is that energy needs vary from day to day. What you eat also varies. So the balance between calories consumed and calories expended is constantly shifting.

Tracking these shifts requires some old-fashioned accounting — tallying up all sources of energy income (what you eat and drink) and all forms of energy expenditure (physical activity). Tracking is helpful in losing weight (and why it's part of *The Mayo Clinic Diet*), but most people don't want to do it forever.

Over the long haul, it's better to think about weight control in terms of general principles — to lose weight you need to eat foods that contain fewer calories and you need to burn more calories through physical activity.

The best way to do this is with practice — eating more fruits, vegetables and whole grains and less fat, and exercising more. Eventually, you'll start doing this on your own without even thinking about it; it will become habit. That's the goal of this book — to help you follow a more healthy lifestyle.

Reducing calories tends to figure more prominently than does physical activity during the initial stages of weight loss. But as you work toward a healthy weight, physical activity is more and more essential to reaching your goal.

Healthy weight control

So, do you need to eat carrots and celery sticks and avoid even the sight of chocolate for the rest of your life in order to maintain a healthy weight?

No. In terms of energy balance, it's possible to eat any food you like and lose weight as long as the total calories you consume are less than the total calories you burn. But what you eat affects your health.

If the bulk of your diet consists of foods that are high in saturated fat, you increase your risk of cardiovascular disease and other diseases. And diets high in refined carbohydrates and low in fiber are linked to conditions such as diabetes and cardiovascular disease. In addition, if your diet is lacking vegetables and fruits, you're missing the health benefits of vitamins and minerals, phytochemicals, and antioxidants.

The science behind it

The everyday decisions you make regarding the food you eat and the activity you do and, ultimately, the weight you carry, relate to what's called the first law of thermodynamics. This law states that energy must remain constant — it's neither created nor destroyed, but merely transferred or converted to different forms.

The calories you eat can either be converted to physical energy or stored within your body, but they can't magically disappear. All unused calories in your body become fat, regardless of where they come from. Unless you use these stored calories, either by reducing calorie intake so that your body must draw on reserves for energy or by increasing physical activity and the amount of energy you expend, this fat will remain in your body.

In theory, the energy balance equation is simple. In practice, applying it can be a bit more complex. But as you grasp the concept of energy balance, weight control may become easier to understand. And a key point is that a healthy weight can be achieved in a way that allows you to enjoy food as well as long-term health.

Understanding energy density

In the next chapter, you'll learn about energy density. Energy density refers to the number of calories in the amount (volume) of food you eat.

Foods with a lot of calories packed into each bite are high in energy density. Those with fewer calories in each bite are low in energy density.

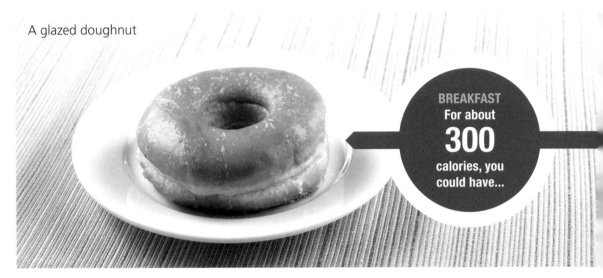

A glazed doughnut

BREAKFAST
For about
300
calories, you could have...

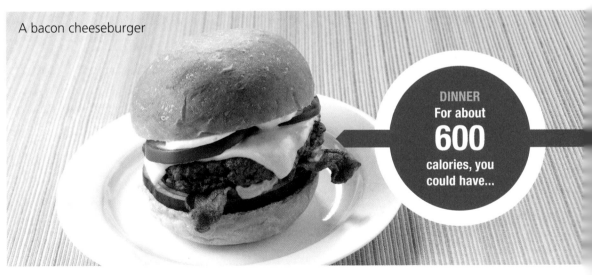

A bacon cheeseburger

DINNER
For about
600
calories, you could have...

By eating foods low in energy density, you can eat more food for less calories. Plus, foods low in energy density are more likely to fill you up. The images below provide a visual comparison. The foods on the left are high-energy-dense foods, while those on the right are low in energy density.

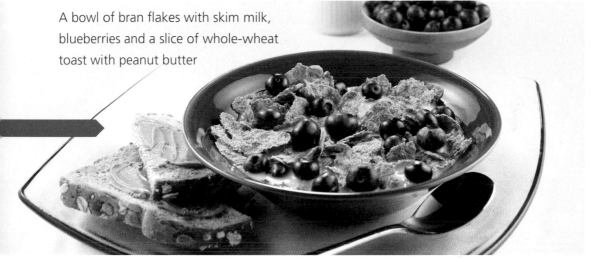

A bowl of bran flakes with skim milk, blueberries and a slice of whole-wheat toast with peanut butter

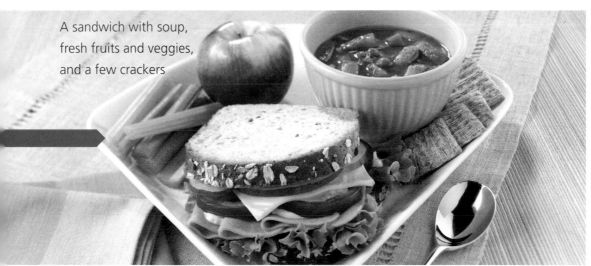

A sandwich with soup, fresh fruits and veggies, and a few crackers

Chapter 15
The Mayo Clinic Healthy Weight Pyramid

In the last chapter, the main theme was *energy*. In this chapter, think *volume*. Combined — as in the amount of energy in a given volume of food — you have *energy density*, the underlying principle of the Mayo Clinic Healthy Weight Pyramid. The concept of energy density is an important weight-loss tool.

If you think about what determines how much food you eat, it generally isn't calories. You don't say to yourself, "I've eaten 500 calories, now I'm full. I'm done eating." You eat until you're satisfied from consuming enough food.

If you eat foods that provide a lot of weight and volume (bulk) but not many calories, you can feel full and still lose weight or maintain your weight. The Mayo Clinic Healthy Weight Pyramid is designed to help you do just that. To lose weight, you shouldn't have to spend your day feeling hungry all of the time.

In addition to weight loss, health is obviously important, which is why the Mayo Clinic Healthy Weight Pyramid emphasizes health-promoting choices within each of its six food groups.

Vegetables and fruits are the foundation of the pyramid. You can eat virtually unlimited amounts of fresh or frozen veggies and fruits (not dried fruits or juices) because of their beneficial effects on both weight and health. Whole-grain carbohydrates, which are healthier than are their refined (think white flour) counterparts, should be eaten in moderate amounts. Protein, dairy and heart-healthy unsaturated fats also are part of a healthy diet, but you need to limit their amounts. Even an occasional treat is OK.

Energy density

All foods contain a certain number of calories (energy) in a given amount (volume), and the number varies from one type of food to another.

Some foods are high in calories, even for a small amount. They're considered high in energy density. These foods include most high-fat foods, simple sugars, alcohol, fast foods, sodas, candies and processed foods. Other foods don't have many calories, even for a relatively large amount. These foods, such as vegetables and fruits, are low in energy density.

Let's consider a couple of examples. A regular candy bar might have 270 calories. A lot of calories in a small package makes for high energy density. In contrast, a cup of raw vegetables contains only about 25 calories. Not many calories in a fairly large volume makes for low energy density. You could eat 11 cups of raw vegetables to get as many calories as you would from that one candy bar.

Where this helps in weight loss is that foods low in energy density typically leave you feeling satisfied on fewer calories, while foods high in energy density are less likely to fill you up — or if you do fill up on them, you've chowed down a lot of calories.

Feeling full on fewer calories may seem like a weight-loss gimmick, but the concept is backed by science. Research suggests that feeling full is strongly determined by the volume and weight of food in your stomach, not necessarily by the number of calories you eat.

Participants in several studies who switched to a diet of low-energy-dense foods were able to lose significant amounts of weight. More importantly, they were able to stick to the low-energy-dense diet and keep much of the weight off over time.

By choosing foods with a low energy density, you can consume fewer calories while still feeling full — and lose weight. That's the heart of the Mayo Clinic Healthy Weight Pyramid.

Now let's look in more detail at the pyramid's individual sections.

Vegetables and fruits

Vegetables and fruits share many attributes. Both offer a wide array of flavors, textures and colors. They provide not only sensory pleasure but also many disease-fighting nutrients.

Most vegetables and fruits are low in energy density because they're high in water and fiber, which provide no calories. You can improve your diet — and actually eat more food — by eating more vegetables and fruits in place of higher calorie foods.

Vegetables

Vegetables include roots and tubers such as carrots, radishes and beets, members of the cabbage family, and salad greens such as lettuce and spinach. Other plant foods, such as tomatoes, peppers and cucumbers, are included in this group, although technically they're fruits.

One pyramid serving of vegetables contains about 25 calories. Vegetables contain no cholesterol, are low in fat and sodium, and are high in dietary fiber. They're also high in essential minerals such as potassium and magnesium and contain beneficial plant chemicals known as phytochemicals.

Fresh vegetables are best, but frozen vegetables are good, too. Most canned vegetables are high in sodium because sodium is used as a preservative in the canning process. If you use canned vegetables, look for labels that indicate that no salt has been added, or rinse them before use.

Fruits

Most foods that contain seeds surrounded by an edible layer are generally considered a fruit. In North America, fruits such as apples, oranges, peaches and plums, and slightly more exotic fruits, such as

Less dense, more filling

Three factors play important roles in what makes vegetables and fruits less energy dense and more filling:

88%
water
52 calories

+ **Water** — Most fruits and vegetables contain a lot of water, which provides volume and weight but not calories. A small grapefruit, for example, is about 90 percent water and has just 64 calories. Carrots are about 88 percent water and have only 52 calories in 1 cup (more than two pyramid servings).
+ **Fat** — Most fruits and vegetables do not contain a lot of fat. Fat raises energy density. One teaspoon of butter contains almost the same number of calories as 2 cups of broccoli!
+ **Fiber** — Fiber is the part of plant-based foods that your body doesn't absorb. The high-fiber content in foods such as vegetables, fruits and whole grains provides bulk to your diet, so it makes you feel full sooner. The fiber also takes longer to digest, making you feel full longer.

mangos and papayas, are commonly available.

Similar to vegetables, fruits are great sources of fiber, vitamins, minerals and other phytochemicals. One pyramid serving equals about 60 calories and is virtually fat-free. Fruits can help you control your weight and reduce your risk of weight-related diseases.

Fresh fruit is best, but frozen fruits with no added sugar and fruits canned in their own juice or water also are excellent. Because of processing, fruit juice and dried fruits, such as raisins and prunes, can be a concentrated source of calories — they have a higher energy density. Eat them sparingly.

Carbohydrates

Carbohydrates include a wide range of foods that are major energy sources for your body. One pyramid serving is about 70 calories. Most carbohydrates are plant based. They include grain products, such as breads, cereals and pasta, and certain starchy vegetables, such as potatoes and corn. Which kind should you focus on?

Think of all the carbohydrate-containing foods laid out in a line. At one end are whole wheat, oats and brown rice. In the middle, white flour, white rice, potatoes and pastas. And at the other end are highly processed products — cookies, candies and soft drinks.

The foods in that spectrum incorporate all three kinds of carbohydrates: fiber, starch and sugar. It's not hard to point to the healthy and less healthy ends — less refined whole grains on one end, highly refined sugar on the other. The health pros and cons of items in the middle aren't so clear. Rice, pasta and bread can all shift depending on how they're processed and served.

Consider, for example, white and whole-wheat (whole-grain) breads. Both begin as nutrient-rich whole grains. During processing, however, the grain's bran and germ are refined away, taking with them many of their vitamins and almost all of their fiber.

When picking carbohydrates, the key word is *whole*. Generally, the less refined a carbohydrate food, the better it is for you.

What if you have diabetes?

You want a snack, and there's an orange handy. But you've been told to limit fruit because you have diabetes, and there are carbs in fruit. You're concerned about what that orange will do to your blood sugar.

What should you do?

That depends on you. If you're overweight and you're closely following the calorie and activity guidelines of this book, you'll lose excess pounds. And if you're losing weight, eating fruit likely won't affect your blood sugar in a negative way.

Chances are, you'll be just fine following the eating guidelines of the Mayo Clinic Healthy Weight Pyramid, which allows unlimited fruits and vegetables. But, you still need to monitor your blood sugar to see how the diet is affecting you.

The Mayo Clinic Healthy Weight Pyramid is suitable for the vast majority of people, including most people with health concerns such as diabetes and high triglycerides. But, as with any valid eating plan, it's not a one-size-fits-all approach. You may need to adapt it to your specific situation. For example, you may do better eating small meals more frequently than three major meals.

The Mayo Clinic Healthy Weight Pyramid has enough flexibility to allow for modifications, so work with your doctor or a registered dietitian to find out how to apply the pyramid to your eating plan in a way that works best for you.

Protein and dairy

Protein is essential to human life. Your skin, bone, muscle and organ tissues are made up of protein, and it's present in your blood, too.

Protein is often associated with foods of animal origin, such as red meat, but it's also found in plants.

Foods rich in protein and relatively low in fat and saturated fat include legumes, fish, skinless poultry and lean meat. Whole-milk dairy products are good sources of protein and calcium, but they're high in saturated fat. Low-fat or skim milk, yogurt, and cheese have the same nutritional value as the whole-milk varieties but without the fat and calories. They're relatively

Gluten-free carbohydrates

If you have a gluten-related disorder such as celiac disease or non-celiac gluten sensitivity, avoiding foods made with gluten is essential to your daily diet. You may wonder if you can follow the diet if you can't eat gluten.

The answer is, yes, you can. There are a number of grains that provide beneficial nutrients and fiber that don't contain gluten. Substituting gluten-free grains for those that contain gluten — wheat, barley and rye — shouldn't affect your diet.

As with other carbohydrates, the key is limiting the amount you eat and selecting from the healthy end of the spectrum. Eat minimally processed foods made from gluten-free whole grains such as buckwheat, quinoa, and brown and wild rice. Avoid processed foods such as gluten-free crackers, chips and cookies.

Many people avoid foods containing gluten because they believe gluten-free foods are healthier, which is not true. If you don't have celiac disease or gluten sensitivity, eating whole grains containing gluten is healthier than not eating them.

low in energy density, too, because they contain a lot of water.

Many cuts of chicken, turkey, beef, lamb and pork can be too high in saturated fat and cholesterol to include regularly in a healthy diet. Focus on lean cuts of meat, and remember that other foods you eat everyday, including low-fat dairy products, seafood and many plant foods, provide protein, too.

Legumes — namely beans, lentils, and peas — are an excellent source of protein because they have no cholesterol and very little fat. They're great for filling out or replacing dishes made with poultry or meat. Unlike meat, beans help lower the "bad" form of cholesterol (LDL), and the minerals they contain help control blood pressure.

Except for soybeans, the protein in beans is "incomplete," meaning it lacks essential amino acids that meats provide, the missing nutrients are plentiful in other plant foods, so people who lighten up on meat can easily get all the protein they need from other foods.

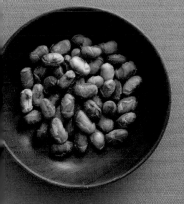

BEST CHOICE
Soy

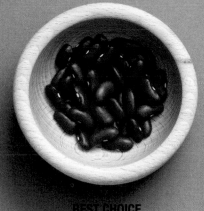

BEST CHOICE
Other beans/peas

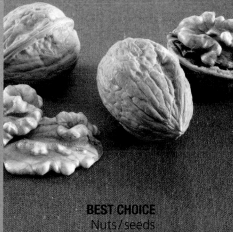

BEST CHOICE
Nuts/seeds

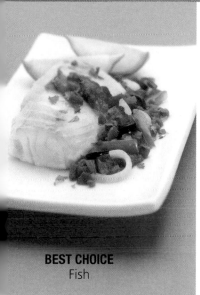

BEST CHOICE
Fish

The protein spectrum

Not all proteins are the same. Some proteins are healthier for you than others. It's good to vary your protein sources, but make sure to eat more healthy proteins and fewer unhealthy ones. Proteins on the lower end of the spectrum contain saturated fat. Red meat and processed meats have been linked to a higher risk of cancer.

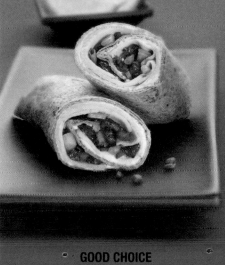

GOOD CHOICE
Chicken/turkey

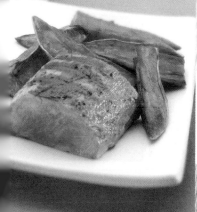

LEAST HEALTHY
Pork

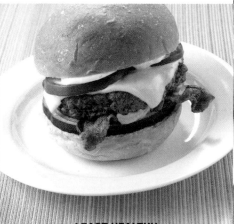

LEAST HEALTHY
Red meat

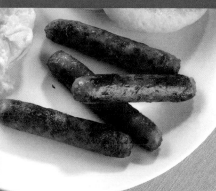

LEAST HEALTHY
Processed meat

Fish and shellfish are not only good protein sources but some types also supply omega-3 fatty acids, which can help lower triglycerides. Triglycerides are fat particles in blood that appear to raise your risk of heart disease. Omega-3 fatty acids may also help prevent heartbeat disturbances known as arrhythmias, improve immune function and help regulate blood pressure.

Research suggests that most people would benefit by eating at least two servings of fish a week. Fatty fish, such as salmon, lake trout, herring, sardines and tuna, contain the most omega-3 fatty acids and therefore the most benefit. But many types of seafood contain small amounts of omega-3 fatty acids.

One serving from the protein and dairy group provides 110 calories.

Fats

Fats are essential to the life and function of your body's cells. Along with providing reserves of stored energy, fats play a role in your immune function, help maintain cell structure and play a role in the regulation of many other body processes. In short, you need some fat in your diet.

But not all fats are created equal (see page 29). Studies indicate that people who replace much of the animal fat in their diets — including solid shortenings and margarines — with canola and olive oils stand a good chance of reducing their blood cholesterol levels and their risk of cardiovascular disease.

A key point: The pyramid's fat group recommendations address only fats that are typically *added* to a day's meals, not the fat within other foods (such as meats). Added fats include salad dressings, cooking oils, butter and high-fat plant foods, such as avocados, olives, seeds and nuts.

Most high-fat plant foods are good for you. Nuts, for instance, contain monounsaturated fat, a type of fat that helps keep your heart and arteries free of harmful deposits. Nuts are also a good source of protein, and depending on the type, may deliver many other key nutrients. But while nuts may be beneficial, they're high in calories. For that reason, all fats should be consumed sparingly.

And what about the fat within meat, seafood and many dairy products? It's limited by way of the serving recommendations for the various pyramid food groups.

Sweets

Foods in the sweets group include sugar-sweetened beverages, candies, desserts, and so on. And don't forget the table sugar you may add to cereal, fruit and beverages.

Because they tend to contain a lot of sugar and fat, sweets are high in energy density and a major source of calories. They also offer little in terms of nutrition. You don't have to give up sweets entirely. But be smart about your selections and portion sizes.

The pyramid recommends limiting sweets to 75 calories a day. For practicality, average that over a week. Where possible, select better dessert choices, such as a small amount of dark chocolate or low-fat frozen yogurt.

Where does alcohol fit?

Alcohol is a fairly concentrated source of calories — about 7 calories per gram (topped only by fat) — but has no nutritional value. For that reason, it's included under sweets in the Mayo Clinic Healthy Weight Pyramid.

Consider it a treat. You don't have to eliminate it under the *Live It!* phase of *The Mayo Clinic Diet*, but limit your consumption to an average of 75 calories a day over the course of a week.

→ For more on alcohol, see page 157.

Physical activity

The Mayo Clinic Healthy Weight Pyramid isn't just about food. The pyramid also recommends 30 to 60 minutes of moderately vigorous physical activity most days of the week.

For more on how to accomplish that, see Chapters 10 and 19.

Chapter 16
Making meals easier

When you eat at home, you typically consume fewer calories. But homemade meals can take time, and it seems there's never have enough of that. In order to have great meals that are tasty and healthy, as well as simple and practical, you need a good process for planning them. This chapter can give you some tips on how to do that.

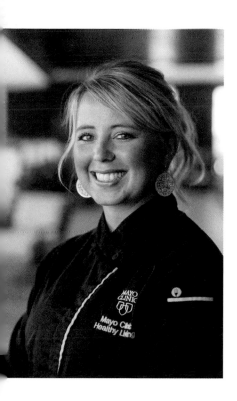

Jennifer A. Welper

Chef, Mayo Clinic
Healthy Living Program

When it comes to cooking healthy, it's important to have a plan that includes a list of meals for the upcoming week. If you don't have some type of plan, meal preparation becomes more difficult and time-consuming, which can make your cooking and eating experience less enjoyable.

Another key to hassle-free meals is learning how to maximize your time and energy in the kitchen. Whenever you're preparing food, think ahead and prep for the week. The more efficient you can be, the less time you need to spend cooking. Then, on busy days or hectic nights, all you need to do is assemble your meals because you've got everything ready to go.

In this chapter, we'll talk about some simple strategies to help make meal preparation less time-consuming and more enjoyable. For example, if you're cutting vegetables for today's soup, cut up some more for tomorrow's pasta salad or roasted vegetables later in the week. If you're baking a chicken breast for dinner and you plan to have a chicken wrap later in the week, prepare another chicken breast at the same time, cool it and place it in fridge.

If this seems overwhelming, start with small steps. If you rarely cook for yourself, start with one or two meals a week and gradually add more. Soon, you'll become more confident in making your own meals. And remember, have fun and don't be afraid to experiment!

Grocery shopping

The recipe to making healthy meals starts in the grocery store. That's because you can't eat — or prepare — what you don't have!

Just like you want to keep foods that can sabotage your weight-loss efforts out of the house, you want to make sure those foods that can aid your efforts are in the house, and in abundance! Here are some basic strategies to ensure that you have the right foods on hand.

1. Plan ahead

Decide how many evening meals you'll be shopping for. Then, consider the food items you'll need for breakfasts, lunches and snacks. Take an inventory of your pyramid essentials, such as fresh fruits and vegetables, whole grains, and low-fat dairy products. See the opposite page for ideas.

As you plan, think about centering the week's meals around a set of core ingredients. If you know you'll be shopping for peppers and onions for fajitas one night, buy some extra peppers and onions for pita pizzas another night. You'll cut down on the time spent shopping for different kinds of foods.

2. Make a list

A list makes your shopping trip more efficient, and it helps you avoid impulse purchases. But don't let your list prevent you from looking for or trying new healthy foods.

When making your list, use your meal plan for the week as your guide. Make sure your list also includes healthy and convenient snack foods.

3. Be intentional

Skip the processed snack foods and sugary beverages aisles. Stick to the sections of your grocery store stocked with the foods on your list — fresh produce, low-fat dairy, and meat and seafood sections.

Remember, fresh foods are generally better than ready-to-eat foods because you can control any ingredients that you add. Aisles stocked with healthy

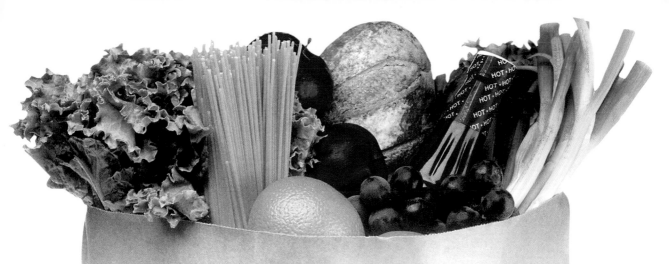

Stock up on these items

Healthy meals can come together in minutes — if you have what you need. When putting together your shopping list, make sure to include the following items:

FRUITS AND VEGETABLES

+ Fresh vegetables
+ Pre-cut fresh vegetables
+ Frozen vegetables (no sauce)
+ Salad in a bag
+ Fresh fruits
+ Canned fruits (packed in their own juice or water)
+ Frozen fruits
+ Fat-free tomato sauce

WHOLE GRAINS

+ Whole-grain breakfast cereal
+ Rice (brown, wild, blends)
+ Oatmeal
+ Whole-grain bread
+ Whole-grain pita bread
+ Whole-grain pasta

PROTEIN

+ Low-fat refried beans
+ Canned black or kidney beans
+ Low-sodium water-packed tuna
+ Other fish with omega-3s
+ Skinless white meat poultry
+ Tofu
+ Natural peanut butter

DAIRY

+ Low-fat or fat-free yogurt
+ Low-fat or fat-free cheese
+ Reduced-fat cream cheese
+ Fat-free or 1% milk

DAIRY-FREE

+ Coconut or soy yogurt
+ Soy, rice or almond milk
+ Dairy-free cheese

What to look for on the nutrition label

❶ Check the serving size

How many servings are in the container?
A serving may be smaller than you think.

❷ Check the calories in one serving

40 calories is low
100 calories is moderate
400 calories or more is high

Nutrition Facts

❶
8 servings per container
Serving size   2/3 cup (55g)

❷
Amount per serving
Calories   230

❸
	% Daily Value*
Total Fat 8g	**10%**
Saturated Fat 1g	**5%**
Trans Fat 0g	
Cholesterol 0mg	**0%**
Sodium 160mg	**7%**
Total Carbohydrate 37g	**13%**
Dietary Fiber 4g	**14%**
Total Sugars 12g	
Includes 10g Added Sugars	**20%**
Protein 3g	
Vitamin D 2mcg	10%
Calcium 260mg	20%
Iron 8mg	45%
Potassium 235mg	6%

* The % Daily Value (DV) tells you how much a nutrient in a serving of food contributes to a daily diet. 2,000 calories a day is used for general nutrition advice.

❸ Check the % Daily Value*

Low is 5% or less. Aim low in saturated fat, trans fat, cholesterol and sodium.
High is 20% or more. Aim high in vitamins, minerals and fiber.

❱❱ Limit nutrients shown in orange
❱❱ Get enough of nutrients shown in green

❹ Check the ingredients

Ingredients are listed by volume. The higher up on the list an ingredient is, the more of it the product contains. Make sure sugar isn't one of the first ingredients listed. Sugar goes by many names, including high-fructose corn syrup, barley malt syrup and dehydrated cane juice, to name a few.

*The % Daily Value (DV) tells you how much a nutrient in a serving of food contributes to a daily diet. 2,000 calories a day is used for general nutrition advice. For the example shown, the recommended goal for dietary fiber is 28 grams, so 4 grams is 14% DV.

Adapted from U.S. Food and Drug Administration, 2016.

❹ INGREDIENTS: ENRICHED FLOUR, (WHEAT FLOUR, CALCIUM GLUCONATE, REDUCED IRON, ASCORBIC ACID, RETINOIC ACID) GRAHAM FLOUR, ORGANIC CANE SUGAR, PARTIALLY HYDROGENATED COTTONSEED OIL, MOLASSES, LEAVENING (SODIUM BICARBONATE), SEA SALT, ARTIFICIAL FLAVOR

items such as oatmeal, beans, whole grains and canned fruits and vegetables are another good place to shop.

4. Don't shop when you're hungry

Let's face it, it's harder to resist buying high-fat, high-calorie snack items when you're hungry. So set yourself up for success and shop after you've eaten a good meal. If you do find yourself shopping on an empty stomach, drink some water or buy a piece of fruit to munch on.

5. Read nutrition labels

Check nutrition labels for serving size, calories, fat, cholesterol and sodium (see the opposite page). Remember, even low-fat and fat-free foods can pack a lot of calories. Compare similar products so that you can choose the healthiest options.

Time-saving strategies

Preparing meals at home doesn't have to eat up all of your time. With some advance planning, you can fit home-made meals into your busy schedule.

Have a plan

Write down your meal plan for the week and stick it on your refrigerator. It can help you organize your time and remember important tasks. Having a plan in front of you every day will keep you on track and motivated.

Combine your prep work

If you're chopping broccoli for a stir fry, chop all the vegetables you'll need for the next few days. Store them in clear containers so that you can easily find them when you need them. The same goes for meat or other proteins. When preparing protein for one dinner, prepare some for the next few meals, too (learn how on page 179).

Another time-saving strategy is to set aside two times each week, including at least one weekend day, to do the majority of your food preparation. At each prep session, work ahead on meals for the next three to four days. Do as much chopping, mixing and cooking as you can. You'll shorten the time you spend in the kitchen the rest of the week.

Overlap ingredients

Save time by planning two meals around similar ingredients. Say you're making brown rice with sautéed carrots, green beans and zucchini. Why not use those same ingredients in a hearty rice soup another night? When preparing the rice and vegetables, make a double batch.

Both meals contain some of the same ingredients but incorporate different flavors and textures. Think about other dishes you enjoy that use overlapping ingredients, and put them on the same weekly menu.

Make extra and freeze it

If you're making a more time-consuming dish for dinner, prepare extra to freeze and heat up later. This works well with many sauces and casseroles.

It's also a good option for individual foods, such as breaded chicken breasts and uncooked pita pizzas. Make the extras and place them on a baking sheet in the freezer. Once they're fully frozen, wrap them in plastic wrap to use later. On another night, unwrap what you need and bake it. For the best flavor and texture, place the item into oven still frozen and bake at a high temperature of 425 to 450 F.

Use your freezer wisely

Freezing extra food can save you a lot of time in the long run — but not if you freeze it and forget it. Make a plan to use any food you're going to freeze. For example, if you freeze several weeks' worth of breaded chicken breasts, plan on using them for one dinner each week over the next month.

A good rule of thumb is to use frozen foods within three months. Clearly date and label them, and keep a list of your freezer's contents. Periodically go through your freezer to remove foods that are unidentifiable or have been sitting in your freezer for too long.

Have a system

Set up a routine around mealtimes. You might make a habit of turning the oven on as soon as you get home from work. Maybe your older child

Shortcuts in the kitchen

Preparing food in bulk can be a time saver. Try some of these tips to reduce your time in the kitchen.

Protein

Prepare two meals' worth of chicken, fish or other lean meat at one time. Use half the protein for tonight's dinner. Place the extra in a shallow container and chill it in the refrigerator for up to three or four days. For any type of meat, reheat it until it reaches a safe internal temperature of 165 F.

Brown rice

Brown rice is flavorful, healthy and filling, but it takes around 50 minutes to cook. To save time, make a large batch. When the rice is done, spread it out on a baking sheet to cool. Then put ½-cup servings or family-sized servings in sealable bags to store in the freezer. To reheat the rice, microwave some water in a bowl or large measuring cup. Soak the rice in the hot water to heat it through, then drain.

Pasta

If you're making pasta for dinner, make extra for later on. You can store the extra pasta in the refrigerator for a week or two. If you made spaghetti with marinara sauce one night, another night toss the extra pasta with a little sesame oil, soy sauce and some stir-fry vegetables to make lo mein.

To measure pasta, take all of the noodles out of a box that says it contains eight servings, divide the noodles into 16 equal portions, and place each of the 16 portions into individual plastic bags. According to Mayo Clinic Health Weight Pyramid serving sizes, one bag equals one serving.

Potatoes

If your menu plan includes potatoes a couple of nights, cut them all at once and store them in containers of cold water in the refrigerator. When you need them, pat them dry, then season and cook them as you normally would.

assembles the prepared dinner ingredients while you help your younger one with homework. Involve the family and make it fun. Cooking together not only gives you a chance to connect, but also teaches healthy skills and habits.

Use dinner ingredients for lunch

Intentionally plan for leftovers. By making enough for two meals at once, you'll save time. Leftovers make a great lunch. If you want a little more variety, use your dinner ingredients in different ways. Take an unused tortilla from your dinner tacos to make a lunch wrap. Slice up an extra piece of grilled chicken breast for a sandwich or Asian chicken salad.

Healthy ways to prepare your food

Healthy cooking doesn't mean you have to become a gourmet chef or invest in special cookware. Simply use standard cooking methods to prepare foods in healthy ways. You can also adapt familiar recipes by substituting other ingredients for fat, sugar and salt (see page 183).

Use these methods

These methods best capture the flavor and retain the nutrients in your food without adding too much fat or salt.

+ **Baking.** Besides breads and desserts, you can bake seafood, poultry, lean meat, and vegetables and fruits that are somewhat uniform in size. Place food in a pan or dish (covered or uncovered) and bake. If you're used to frying foods, baking is a good alternative.

+ **Grilling and broiling.** Both grilling and broiling expose fairly thin pieces of food to direct heat and allow fat to drip away from the food. If you're grilling outdoors, place smaller items, such as chopped vegetables, in a long-handled grill basket or on foil to prevent pieces from slipping through the rack. To broil indoors, place food on a broiler rack below a heat element.

+ **Roasting.** Roasting uses an oven's dry heat at high temperatures to cook food placed on a baking sheet or in a roasting pan. Like baking, this is a good option if you're trying to avoid frying. For poultry, seafood and meat, place a rack inside the roasting pan so that the fat can drip away during cooking. Roasted vegetables also are a tasty addition to a healthy meal. Toss them with a small amount of oil or coat a baking sheet with cooking spray before adding the vegetables.

+ **Sautéing.** Sautéing cooks small or thin pieces of food in a shallow pan. If you choose a good-quality nonstick pan, such as a hard anodized pan, you can cook food without much fat. Heat the pan on high heat for a few minutes before cooking. Once you add the food, stir it about every 30 seconds. Depending on the recipe, use low-sodium broth, cooking spray, water or wine in place of oil or butter. For sautéing, searing and stir-frying, hard anodized cookware is best because you can use small amounts of oil.

+ **Searing.** Searing quickly browns the surface of food at a high temperature. It locks in flavor and adds a crusty texture to meats and other proteins. Heat a pan on high heat and use a small amount of oil for a golden crust. This method works well with all types of meat, including poultry, fish and lean beef. Some plant-based proteins such as tofu and tempeh also can be seared.

+ **Stir-frying.** Stir-frying is similar to sautéing but cooks food more quickly. It works best with small, uniform-sized pieces of food that are rapidly and continuously stirred in a wok or large nonstick frying pan. You need only a small amount of oil or cooking spray for this cooking method.

+ **Steaming.** One of the simplest cooking techniques to master is steaming food in a perforated basket or bamboo basket suspended above simmering liquid. Steaming can be used for a variety of vegetables, as well as tender meats such as fish and poultry. If you use a flavorful liquid or add herbs to the water, you'll flavor the food as it cooks.

New ways to flavor food

Instead of salt or butter, you can enhance foods with a variety of herbs, spices and low-fat condiments such as vinegars, citrus juices, and low-sodium marinades or sauces. Don't be afraid to be creative.

For example, you can top a broiled chicken breast with fresh salsa. You can also make meats more flavorful with low-fat marinades or spices — bay leaf, chili powder, dry mustard, garlic, ginger, cayenne pepper, cumin, sage, marjoram, onion, oregano, pepper or thyme. On page 187 you'll find recipes for handy rubs to enhance the flavor of your foods.

Canola and olive oils are some of your healthiest options when it comes to preparing seafood, chicken and meat or dressings for salads. To change up the flavor, try adding a small amount of savory oils to your dishes. Coconut oil and oils made from nuts and seeds — such as walnut and sesame oil — can add an extra dimension of flavor. Add a little to your pan, or sprinkle some on salads or cooked dishes.

Another way to enhance dressings, marinades, fresh vegetables and cooked dishes, is to add a splash of flavorful vinegar, such as balsamic, wine or rice vinegar.

To bring out the flavor in baked goods, use a bit more vanilla, cinnamon or nutmeg rather than more sugar.

Learning to mix and match

It's easy when cooking to get caught in a rut. We tend to make the same things over and over again. Often, the problem is, we don't know how to mix things up!

You don't need to purchase a lot of food or ingredients to mix and match your meals. Here are some tips on how to combine different foods and ingredients to get out of that rut.

Mix-and-match meals

There's no right or wrong way to combine these meal options. Experiment, and let your taste buds lead the way. You might discover some new favorites!

Adapting recipes

If the recipe calls for	Try substituting
Butter Margarine Shortening Oil	✚ For sandwiches, substitute tomato slices, ketchup or mustard. ✚ For stove-top cooking, sauté food in broth or small amounts of healthy oil such as olive, canola or peanut or use cooking spray. ✚ In marinades, substitute diluted fruit juice, wine or balsamic vinegar. ✚ In cakes or bars, replace half the fat or oil with the same amount of fat-free plain yogurt, prune purée or commercial fat substitute. ✚ To avoid dense, soggy or flat baked goods, don't substitute oil for butter or shortening, or substitute diet, whipped or tub-style margarine for regular margarine.
Meat	Keep it lean. In soup, chili or stir-fry, replace most of the meat with beans or vegetables. As an entree, keep it to no more than the size of a deck of cards — load up on vegetables.
Whole milk (regular or evaporated)	Fat-free or 1% milk, or evaporated skim milk.
Whole egg (yolk and white)	¼ cup egg substitute or 2 egg whites for breakfast or in baked goods.
Sour cream Cream cheese	Fat-free, low-fat or light varieties in dips, spreads, salad dressings and toppings. Fat-free, low-fat and light varieties may not work as well for baking.
Sugar	In most baked goods, you can reduce the amount of sugar by one-half without affecting texture or taste, but use no less than ¼ cup of sugar for every cup of flour to keep items moist.
White flour	Replace half or more of white flour with whole-grain pastry or regular flour.
Salt	✚ Use herbs (1 tbsp. fresh = 1 tsp. dried = ¼ tsp. powder). Add toward the end of cooking and use sparingly. You can always add more. ✚ Salt is required when baking yeast-leavened items. Otherwise you may reduce salt by half in cookies and bars. Not needed when boiling pasta.

See the chart on the opposite page. It offers suggestions on how you can combine different meats and seafood with different sauces. Add on a carbohydrate and vegetable serving and you have a meal. Here are a few examples to get you started:

+ **Night 1.** Grill a chicken breast and coat it in a small amount of BBQ sauce. Serve it with a baked potato and grilled asparagus.

+ **Night 2.** Make meatballs made with ground turkey breast. When cooked, cover the meatballs in marinara sauce. Place them over whole-wheat pasta and roasted Brussels sprouts or zucchini.

+ **Night 3.** Sauté some shrimp and drizzle with teriyaki sauce. Serve them with stir-fried peppers, carrots and broccoli over brown rice.

+ **Night 4.** Prepare tacos made from ground lean beef. Place the meat mixture in a whole-wheat tortilla and cover with lettuce, tomatoes, onions and peppers.

+ **Night 5.** Sear or grill some tuna, topped with sweet mango salsa. Serve it with oven-baked sweet potato fries and steamed carrots and green beans.

Mix-and-match salads

Having a salad is a great way to include more vegetables and fruits in your diet. You might think of a salad as some lettuce and tomatoes topped with croutons and dressing. A salad can be a lot more than that, and there are plenty of ways to prepare a healthy and tasty salad.

The next time you have a salad, don't be afraid to experiment. See the chart on page 186. To prepare a nutritious and tasty salad, pick one or more ingredients from each column.

For example, you might have some arugula and leaf lettuce, topped with black beans, tomatoes, cucumbers, orange bell peppers, sunflower seeds and grated Parmesan cheese, and sprinkled with balsamic vinegar and olive oil.

Try 1 of these meats	with 1 of these sauces	plus 1 of these carbohydrates	and a large portion of vegetables
Beef tenderloin **Chicken breast** **Ground lean beef** **Ground pork tenderloin** **Ground turkey breast** **Pork tenderloin** **Turkey breast**	+ BBQ + Hoisin + Marinara + Marsala + Teriyaki	+ Brown rice + Brown rice pilaf + Butternut squash + Mashed or baked potatoes with the skin on + Multigrain or whole-wheat pasta + Oven-baked potato fries or sweet potatoes fries + Sweet potatoes with the skin on + Whole-wheat bread + Whole-wheat couscous + Whole-wheat tortillas	+ Asparagus + Bean sprouts + Beets + Bell peppers + Broccoli + Brussels sprouts + Cabbage + Carrots + Cauliflower + Cucumbers + Eggplant + Green beans + Lettuce + Mushrooms + Parsnips + Peas + Snow peas + Spinach + Sugar snap peas + Summer squash + Turnips + Zucchini

Try this seafood	with 1 of these sauces		
Cod **Halibut** **Salmon** **Scallops** **Sea bass** **Shrimp** **Tilapia** **Tuna**	+ Fat-free Italian dressing + Lemon dill + Scampi + Sesame ginger + Sweet and sour mango or pineapple salsa + Teriyaki + White wine		

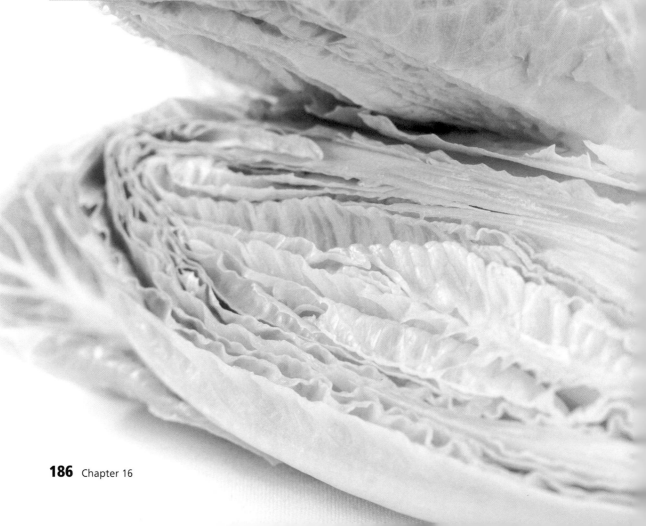

Try 1 of these greens	with 1 of these veggies	plus 1 of these proteins	plus 1 of these toppings	and 1 of these dressings
Arugula **Baby kale** **Bibb lettuce** **Cabbage** **Leaf lettuce** **Romaine** **Spinach** **Spring mix**	✛ Artichokes ✛ Beets ✛ Bell peppers ✛ Broccoli ✛ Carrots ✛ Cauliflower ✛ Cucumbers ✛ Mushrooms ✛ Onions ✛ Peas ✛ Radishes ✛ Tomatoes	✛ Black beans ✛ Chicken breast ✛ Edamame ✛ Extra-firm tofu ✛ Garbanzo beans ✛ Hard-boiled eggs ✛ Kidney beans ✛ Lean ground beef ✛ Salmon ✛ Shrimp ✛ Turkey breast	✛ Croutons ✛ Dried fruit ✛ Fruit ✛ Hard or sharp cheese ✛ Nuts ✛ Seeds	✛ Balsamic vinegar ✛ Cilantro lime ✛ Light Caesar ✛ Light Italian ✛ Low-fat ranch ✛ Low-fat raspberry vinaigrette ✛ Olive oil ✛ Other vinegars ✛ Salsa or taco sauce

Rubbing in flavor

Here are recipes for some basic rubs you can use to flavor meats, seafood and even vegetables.

Herb rub

2 tbsp.	chopped fresh thyme
2 tbsp.	chopped fresh rosemary
2 tbsp.	chopped fresh parsley
1 tbsp.	minced fresh garlic
1 tbsp.	onion powder
1 tbsp.	salt
1 tbsp.	olive oil

Combine the ingredients in a medium bowl. Place the rub mixture on the meat of your choice. Sear the meat on each side, about 2 to 4 minutes, then reduce heat and continue to cook until it reaches the proper internal temperature. Best with chicken, beef or pork.

Souvlaki rub

2 tbsp.	olive oil
1 tbsp.	minced garlic
1 tbsp.	minced fresh oregano
1 tsp.	kosher salt
$\frac{1}{2}$ tsp.	ground black pepper

Combine the ingredients and rub the mixture onto meat or seafood before preparing it, or coat vegetables with the rub before roasting them.

BBQ rub

$\frac{1}{3}$ c.	paprika
$\frac{1}{4}$ c.	brown sugar
2 tbsp.	ground black pepper
2 tbsp.	salt
2 tsp.	dry mustard
2 tsp.	cayenne pepper

This rub can be made in advance and stored in an airtight container. Best used with pork, beef and chicken.

Italian herb rub

2 tbsp.	dried basil
2 tbsp.	dried oregano
1 tbsp.	garlic powder
1 tbsp.	onion powder
1 tsp.	ground fennel
1 tsp.	salt
$\frac{1}{4}$ tsp.	pepper

This rub also can be made in advance. Best used with chicken, lamb, pork tenderloin and vegetables.

Chapter 17
Eating out

Eating out is convenient, efficient, sometimes essential — and let's face it, fun. But the more you eat out, the more likely you are to gain weight. By adopting a few healthy habits, you can enjoy eating out without packing on extra pounds. It's all about being savvy when making decisions.

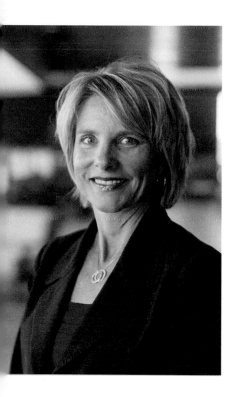

Kristine R. Schmitz, RDN
Clinical Nutrition

Americans like to eat out. And as a nation, we're eating out more than ever — four to five times a week!

According to recent information from the U.S. Department of Commerce, Americans spend more money at restaurants these days than they do at grocery stores. That isn't good for your health, or your waistlines. That's because you're less likely to make healthy choices when you eat out than when you're eating at home.

Recent data show that an average meal at a chain restaurant contains approximately 1,300 calories. If your daily calorie goal is 1,200 calories, one meal at a chain restaurant can provide more calories than you should consume for an entire day.

It's unrealistic to say that you should never eat out. Eating out is fun, and it's convenient. But we would all benefit if we didn't eat out as much as we do. Make it a treat — and look for ways to eat healthfully when you do. Instead of the typical 1,300 calories, aim for a meal that contains fewer calories. Many chain restaurants are now required to list the calorie content of their meals, so choosing wisely has become a bit easier.

In this chapter, we offer tips and suggestions on how to make good food choices when eating away from home. You'll find that you can eat sensibly and still fully enjoy your meal!

Yes, you can dine away from home without sabotaging your weight-loss plan. But you need to play it smart. Just because you're dining out doesn't mean the rules you follow at home don't apply. But it also doesn't mean you're in for an unenjoyable experience. Even when you're trying to lose some weight, you can still savor a tasty meal and have a good time when eating out.

And remember, eating out applies to more than just restaurants. No matter if you're in a coffee shop, buying food at a convenience store, or attending an office potluck or catered event, you're still eating out! As always, selecting the right foods to eat is key.

Plan ahead

When it comes to eating out, being prepared can make all the difference. Set yourself up for success before you even step out the door.

Consider your options. If you don't have a lot of time, it may seem easiest to go to a fast-food restaurant, but remember there are other options.

You can stop at a convenience store and pick up some fruit, a prepackaged salad or a small sandwich. If you have time for a more relaxed meal, stop at a restaurant that has low-calorie options and plenty of fruits and vegetables on the menu.

Go online. Review the menus at restaurants you're considering. When you get to the restaurant it may be hard to study what's available. When you're online, you can check out which restaurants have offerings that fit with your meal plan. You can even look up nutrition information at some restaurant chains. If the calories are posted, consider a meal that provides about 500 to 600 calories. Also check to see if they have low-calorie appetizers or healthy sides.

Have a snack first. If you're meeting friends for a late dinner, eat something an hour or two before you leave. That way, you won't show up famished and be tempted to order more food than you need. You'll also be less likely to fill up on the chips and salsa or bread rolls that sit at the table before your meal arrives.

Plan for the day. If you know you'll be eating out for one meal, eat lighter at your other meals.

Don't eat on the go. Even if your day is packed, take a few minutes to sit down and eat. If you're eating while you're driving, you're more likely to eat too much too quickly and make unhealthy food choices. (It's hard to eat a salad when you're hands are on the wheel!) The end result: You feel guilty and frustrated afterward.

Eating at fast-food restaurants

Fast-food restaurants are everywhere, and they're popular. Among other things, they offer a meal in a hurry when you don't have much time.

But eating at fast-food restaurants on a regular basis isn't a good idea. Perhaps the biggest reasons why are because fast food is often loaded with calories and the portions are often very large. This doesn't mean an occasional stop at a fast-food restaurant is out of the question. Just be smart in what you eat.

Fortunately, making healthy choices at fast-food and other chain restaurants is now easier. The Food and Drug Administration has established new regulations for nutrition labeling in chain restaurants (see pages 192 and 193).

All fast-food and sit-down restaurant chains with at least 20 locations are required to provide nutrition information about the foods they serve on their menus or menu boards. These regulations also apply to drive-thru windows, and to foods sold in bakeries and coffee shops, and many vending machines.

Uncovering clues

No matter where you eat — at a fast-food restaurant or a traditional sit-down restaurant — look for clues (words) on the menu that provide hints about how a food has been prepared.

Certain words such as *breaded*, *creamy* or *fried* are pretty good indicators that calories are added during preparation. Instead, look for *grilled*, *baked* or *steamed*.

What to eat, and not to eat

The next time you stop at a fast-food restaurant, pay attention to the calorie listings. Taking a few minutes to compare the items on the menu can really pay off. Look at these examples (and the calorie amounts) from some of the most popular chains.

McDonald's

Buttermilk crispy chicken sandwich (580) with large french fries (510)	vs.	Artisan grilled chicken sandwich (380) with fruit and yogurt parfait (150)
Total: 1,090 calories		Total: 530 calories

Subway

Foot-long meatball marinara (960) with potato chips (230) and cookie (210)	vs.	6-inch Veggie Delite (230) with bowl of corn chowder (150) and apple slices (35)
Total: 1,400 calories		Total: 415 calories

Burger King

Double Whopper with cheese (930) and vanilla milkshake (580)	vs.	Garden grilled chicken salad with Tender-grill, no dressing (320) and 20-ounce sweet tea (120)
Total: 1,510 calories		Total: 440 calories

Starbucks

20-ounce (venti) white chocolate mocha with fat-free milk (440) and whipped cream (70)	vs.	12-ounce (tall) vanilla latte with fat-free milk and no whipped cream
Total: 510 calories		Total: 150 calories

Olive Garden

Shrimp Alfredo (1,150) with 2 breadsticks with garlic butter spread (280)	vs.	Herb-grilled salmon (460) and house salad with low-fat dressing (100)
Total: 1,430 calories		Total: 560 calories

Chili's

Smothered carnitas burrito with rice (1,090) and black beans (120)	vs.	Pasilla chile chicken (420) with asparagus and garlic roasted tomatoes (70)
Total: 1,210 calories		Total: 490 calories

Applebee's

Bourbon Street steak with side (700) and loaded baked potato (460)	vs.	Pepper-crusted sirloin and whole grains (380) with steamed broccoli (90)
Total: 1,160 calories		Total: 470 calories

Source: Nutrition information from McDonald's, Subway, Burger King, Starbucks, Olive Garden, Chili's, Applebee's, 2016.

Ingredients added to dishes while they're being prepared — for example, oil or butter for cooking — can add hidden calories. So can other ingredients used to enhance the flavor, color or texture of food, such as sauces, toppings or dressings.

The problem is, you may not be aware of these hidden calories. That's why people who eat out a lot often have problems losing weight. They think they're eating something healthy, but they're not aware of all of the hidden calories.

Also watch out for buzzwords. These words paint a picture of a meal that may sound healthy but may actually be packed with hidden calories. Some examples of buzzwords include *gourmet* or *house-made.*

If you're unsure how a menu item is prepared or what ingredients it might contain, ask the server or chef.

Dealing with all the extras

When you eat out, especially at a sit-down restaurant, sometimes selecting your main entrée is only half the battle. What about all of the extra food that comes before, after or with your meal? Even if you order something healthy, you can get waylaid by the other choices you have to make.

+ **Appetizers.** If you have an appetizer, avoid fried or breaded items, which are generally high in calories. Choose an appetizer that contains primarily vegetables, fruit or fish. Fresh fruit and shrimp cocktail served with lemon are good choices.

+ **Soup.** The best choices are broth-based or tomato-based soups. Creamed soups, chowders and puréed soups are generally higher in calories.

+ **Bread.** Muffins, garlic toast and croissants have more fat and calories than do whole-grain bread, breadsticks and crackers. Skip the temptation by asking the server not to bring the breadbasket.

+ **Salad.** Your best choice is a lettuce or spinach salad with a vinaigrette or low-fat dressing on the side.

Your eating out guide

Instead of ordering	Order
Fried, breaded or battered food	+ Grilled + Baked + Broiled without butter + Roasted + Steamed + Poached
French fries, onion rings or other fried side dishes	+ Steamed vegetables + Salad in vinaigrette dressing + Fresh fruit
Alfredo or other creamy sauces	+ Tomato-based or wine-based sauces
Creamy salad dressings	+ Vinegar and oil dressings
Creamy soups	+ Soups in clear broth with vegetables + Tomato or other vegetable-based soups
Mayonnaise, butter, sour cream and tartar sauce	+ Mustard + Lemon or lime juice + Herbs and spices + Pepper + Salsa
Sweetened beverages	+ Water with a lemon slice + Low-fat or skim milk + Unsweetened tea or coffee
A mixed, alcoholic drink	+ Wine + Light beer
Cake, pie, cheesecake or ice cream	+ Sherbet or sorbet + Small sugar cookie + Small piece of angel food cake

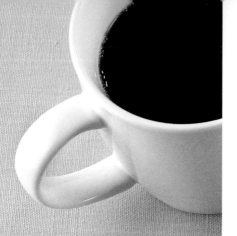

What about that coffee?

When you're trying to limit calories, a plain cup of coffee is a great option. It has only 2 calories — and no fat. The trouble is, it seems fewer people are drinking plain coffee these days. Coffee shops now offer many types of coffee drinks that contain a lot of extras. And these extras — even just a tablespoon's worth — can quickly add up:

+ Heavy whipping cream: 51 calories
+ Table sugar: 49 calories
+ Half-and-half: 18 calories
+ Fat-free milk: 5 calories

When you're at your local coffee shop, check out the nutrition information before you order. Some coffee drinks are more like dessert and can have hundreds of calories. Occasional indulgence is fine. But remember that when it comes to weight loss, all calories count — even calories in liquid form.

Limit all of the high-calorie add-ons, such as cheese and croutons. Mayonnaise-based salads, such as potato salad or macaroni salad, are typically higher in calories. (For more salad tips, see page 198.)

+ **Side dish.** Choose steamed vegetables, fresh fruit, brown rice, a baked potato or boiled new potatoes instead of higher calorie options such as french fries, onion rings and potato chips.

+ **Condiments.** Ask for condiments on the side so that you can control how much you use on your food. Limit high-fat, creamy sauces such as mayonnaise and butter. Some good alternatives are mustard, relish, pepper, salsa, and lemon or lime juice.

+ **Drinks.** Soft drinks, sweet coffee drinks and alcohol-containing beverages can quickly add calories to any restaurant experience. Choose something without calories, such as water or unsweetened tea or coffee. If you do order an alcoholic drink, avoid sweet mixed drinks, which are higher in calories. For more details about the calories in wine, beer and hard liquor, see page 157.

+ **Dessert.** Finish your main meal before ordering dessert. By the time you're done, you may not even want dessert. If you do order dessert, consider splitting it with one of your companions. Some healthy dessert options include sorbet or sherbet.

More helpful strategies

Eating out typically leads to other common challenges. Among them are the urge to order more food than you need and the impulse to eat every bit of food on your plate — even when portion sizes are way too large for one meal.

Unfortunately, large portions have become the norm in most restaurants. People like receiving larger portions because they feel they're getting their money's worth. The trouble is, if you're served more, you generally eat more — even though you often feel just as satisfied eating less.

Plus, if you think that what you're eating is healthy, you may eat even more! Remember, just because you're eating a grilled chicken sandwich doesn't mean it's OK to supersize it.

Here are some strategies to help control how much you eat when you eat out.

Sit-down restaurants

+ **Find an ally.** If one of your dining companions also is trying to eat healthy, sit next to that person.

+ **Make the server your partner.** Don't be afraid to ask for help in managing your meal — like bringing condiments on the side or substituting steamed broccoli for onion rings.

+ **Ask about serving sizes.** Some restaurants offer half-sized or small portions of an entree. Sometimes they're listed as the lunch portion. Don't assume they're too small. And even if they do seem small, you'll likely still feel satisfied when you're done.

¶¶ Eat smart at the salad bar

Whether you're at a buffet, your local grocery store or a sit-down restaurant, you may think that eating at the salad bar is the healthiest option. Yes and no. If you make careful choices, it may be. But if you fill your plate with high-calorie and high-fat foods, you'll end up with more than you bargained for.

+ **Go green.** Lettuce, mixed greens or fresh spinach is generally the foundation of a healthy salad.

+ **Survey the fresh fruits and vegetables.** Pile on fresh vegetables and fruits, such as tomatoes, carrots, broccoli, cauliflower, cucumbers, radishes, bell peppers, pineapple, cantaloupe, watermelon, grapes and strawberries.

+ **Limit the extras.** Many people go wrong at salad bars by including too many high-calorie ingredients. Limit cheese, bacon bits and buttery croutons. Skip creamy pasta salads or potato salad.

+ **Be careful of the dressings.** Select fat-free or low-fat, low-calorie dressings, such as low-fat Italian or reduced-calorie French. Other good options include vinegars.

+ **Check before adding salt or condiments.** You might discover the food is plenty flavorful without adding anything to it.

+ **Eat your sides first.** Order vegetables or fruit as your sides and eat those foods first, before you start in on your entree. By filling up on your sides, you may eat less of your entree, which likely is higher in calories.

+ **Pay attention to the plate.** Plates used at restaurants are often larger than what you use at home. Eat only as much food as would fit easily on an average-sized plate.

+ **Ask for a carryout container.** Ask your server to take away your plate as soon as you feel full. If you have leftovers, take them home for another meal. Better yet, ask that half your meal be boxed-up before it even arrives at the table.

+ **Enjoy the company.** Make an extra effort to focus on the conversation. You may find that you eat more slowly — and eat less.

Fast-food restaurants

+ **Look for the 'light' or 'healthy' section.** You're more likely to find lower-calorie choices, including fruits and vegetables, in this section of the menu.

+ **Don't supersize it.** Avoid oversized items. They can be nearly double the calories of a small order.

+ **Go for grilled.** Seek out grilled meat rather than breaded or fried options. For example, a grilled chicken sandwich can have one-third fewer calories than a crispy chicken sandwich.

+ **Ask for substitutions.** If ordering a combination meal, ask if you can substitute a side salad for the french fries. If not, avoid combo meals and order the items separately.

Buffet or potluck

+ **Survey the offerings.** Rather than jump into the line, first see what's available. By taking this extra time at the start, you'll be more likely to choose well when you select food for your plate.

+ **Have a plan.** Decide ahead of time what you're going to eat and stick with your plan.

+ **Focus on fruits and vegetables.** Fill half your plate with fruits and vegetables. Then pick out a few other things you'd like to try that look healthy or appear somewhat healthy.

+ **Build a colorful plate.** A plate with a variety of colors tends to have a variety of fruits and vegetables.

+ **Use a small dish.** Select a small plate or bowl instead of a large one.

+ **Don't pile it on.** Leave a little room between items to keep your portion sizes in check.

+ **Make one trip.** Plan on just one visit to the buffet line. You may find that it helps to sit at a table that's away from the buffet.

Your guide to healthy ethnic cuisine

Restaurants that specialize in ethnic foods tend to serve large portions, so plan on sharing an entree or taking half of it home.

Here are some other suggestions to help you savor the exotic, while keeping calories, fat and cholesterol under control.

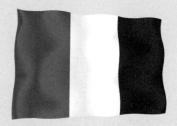

Italian

+ **Go for tomato-based sauces.** Avoid dishes with creamy sauces, such as Alfredo. Opt instead for tomatoes with garlic and onions (marinara), sauces based in wine (Marsala) or sauces cooked with tomatoes, herbs and sometimes wine (cacciatore). Another good option may be pasta primavera with fresh vegetables.

+ **Limit the cheese.** A little cheese adds flavor and texture to your meal, but too much will load up your plate with unwanted calories.

+ **Stay away from high-fat meats.** Avoid dishes containing fat-laden proteins, such as sausage.

+ **Avoid stuffed pasta.** It's usually packed with cheese or fatty meat.

+ **Choose soup.** Opt for vegetable-based soups, such as pasta fagioli or minestrone.

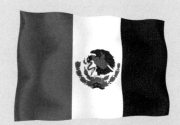

Mexican

+ **Skip the chips.** About 20 chips and 2 tablespoons of salsa contains up to 300 calories.

+ **Steer clear of fried entrees.** Avoid fried foods such as chalupa and chimichanga.

+ **Choose tacos.** Tacos are a smart choice because the shells are often smaller than other nonfried Mexican entrees, such as burritos and enchiladas. Plan on ordering about two tacos. Be adventurous and try a fish or bean taco.

+ **Don't clean your plate.** Entrees at Mexican restaurants are often served on oversized plates with rice and beans. One cup of rice and ½ cup refried beans can add nearly 400 calories to your meal. Take half your dish home.

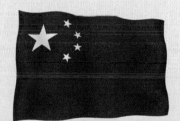

Chinese

+ **Opt for stir-fry.** Choose stir-fried dishes with lots of vegetables. If you order meat, it shouldn't be breaded. Ask to have it prepared with little or no oil, and limit yourself to one portion — an amount that fits easily on a 10-inch plate.

+ **Select steamed rice.** Fried rice is prepared with oil, adding fat and calories to your meal.

+ **Avoid fried appetizers.** Go for spring rolls or steamed dumplings rather than fried appetizers such as egg rolls or fried wontons.

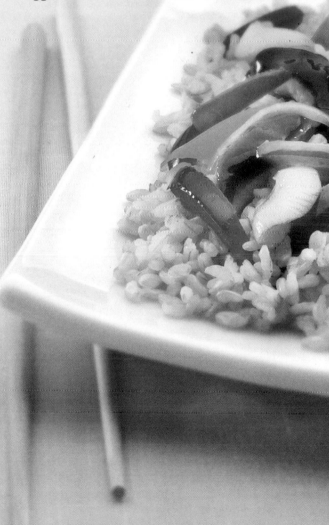

Chapter 18
How to change behaviors

Newborn babies are remarkably direct about food. When they're hungry, they cry. When they're full, they refuse to eat. You probably don't act that way now. Chances are, over time you've learned eating habits in response to factors other than hunger, factors often triggered by a preoccupied brain rather than an empty stomach. But you can change those habits and learn new behaviors.

By being here at this moment and reading this book, you're taking a big step toward a lifelong commitment to healthy living. You're traveling down your wellness journey — a journey of successes and challenges as well as self-discovery.

Anticipate obstacles on this journey. That's because life happens. Even the most thought-out plans for behavior change usually require some adjustments along the way.

But an occasional "off" day doesn't mean failure. It simply means that you get back on track and face tomorrow with renewed confidence in your ability to be successful.

Be realistic with what's ahead of you. It took months or even years to form your current behaviors, so why should you think that you can change those behaviors overnight?

You're striving to make permanent lifestyle changes, and that's no easy task. It will take an adequate amount of time for your new habits to feel natural.

Support and encourage of yourself along the way, and don't forget to reward yourself. No matter how small your achievements, every success is a victory. The journey is yours to succeed at, so enjoy!

Strengthening your resolve

Unfortunately, many people stay on a diet for only a week or two before giving up. Often, this is because they were unable to change their unhealthy behaviors, and their commitment soon weakened. They may have been unable to resist their favorite high-calorie foods. They may have been too tired or too busy to exercise after work. Or they may have struggled to set and track weekly goals.

To achieve and maintain a healthy weight, you need to identify unhealthy behaviors and work to change them permanently. That takes commitment. That takes motivation.

To help strengthen your resolve, before you take specific steps to try and change your behaviors, review the motivators in *Lose It!*

Preparing for change

The only proven formula for achieving and maintaining a healthy weight — eat less and move more — sounds simple. But anyone who's tried to lose weight knows that it's more challenging than it sounds.

Why is that? What gets in the way? Often, it's learned behaviors.

To lose weight, you also need to target key underlying factors, not just what you eat or do. Emotions, social pressure, conditioned thinking, lack of awareness, physical symptoms and other factors influence behaviors.

Changing these ingrained behaviors is a highly individualized process. The method, timing and pace of change vary from one person to the next.

As you contemplate making important changes in your life, here are some general principles to help guide you:

+ **It's not a race.** Sometimes, a little shock therapy can help you think and act differently. That's what's

behind *Lose It!* Those first two weeks are designed to bump you off your normal course and show you that change can bring results.

But long-term lifestyle change typically doesn't happen overnight. It takes time and dedication to unlearn unhealthy behaviors and develop new, healthy ones that can lead to permanent weight loss. Plan for long-term weight loss, but feel free to repeat *Lose It!* if you need a boost and a reminder that change works.

+ **Don't overreact to the scale.** Weighing yourself regularly can help in weight loss, but don't let daily variations in your weight upset you. They may be just fluid changes. You have better control over what you eat and what you do than over numbers on the scale, so concentrate on those actions as your goal.

+ **Anticipate a lapse.** There will be days when you eat more or move less than you intended. This is what's called a lapse, and it's inevitable that you'll occasionally lapse. But it's important not to use a lapse as an excuse to give up. Have a plan for such occasions. See Chapter 20 for more on lapses.

Changing your behaviors

Behavior change doesn't happen by accident. If you want to make lasting changes to your eating and activity habits, you need a plan.

There are many strategies for how to adopt healthier behaviors. Everyone has his or her own approach and his or her own pace for making changes. And it's likely that you won't follow the same plan for every change you want to make. What's important is that you clearly identify and examine the behaviors that interfere with your ability to lose weight and find healthy ways to deal with them.

Here's a list of steps that you may take to change an unhealthy behavior:

1. **List those behaviors that you feel are unhealthy.** Common examples include eating too quickly, snacking throughout the day instead of eating regular meals, eating when you're under stress, and skipping your walk when the weather's not perfect or if the television beckons.

2. **Select one behavior that you would like to change.** Trying to change all the behaviors on your list at once can feel overwhelming and increase the chance that you won't be successful. Focus on changing one behavior at a time.

3. **As you think of strategies for change, consider how you developed the behavior.** Are there underlying causes for the behavior that also need to be addressed? For example, is your all-day snacking related to constant stress? What benefit do you get from the behavior? Are there healthier ways to obtain this benefit? What are the negative consequences of this behavior? Identifying these factors can help outline the reasons for change.

4. **Brainstorm ways to change this behavior.** Think of five to seven possible solutions, then decide on

Put the brakes on stress

Stress can take a toll on your health, cause weight gain and create sleep troubles — all of which can lead to even more stress and derail your weight-loss plans. To stay on track through stressful times, try this four-step strategy:

1. **Take stock of your stressors.** When you're feeling overwhelmed or upset, jot down the particular circumstances in a journal or notebook. **JOT IT** ▶ Realize that stress can be caused by external factors — environment, family relations or unpredictable events — as well as by internal factors — negative attitudes, unrealistic expectations or perfectionism.

2. **Examine your stressors.** Try to identify the problem at its root. Then ask yourself, "Can I change this situation?" or "Can I improve my ability to cope with this situation?" For example, if you always find yourself stressed when deciding what to wear to certain social events, ask yourself why that is. Is it because you don't like your clothes or because you're worried about how someone or some group will judge you? Once you know what's at the root of your stress, you can take steps to deal with it.

3. **Evaluate your responsibilities.** Are you overcommitted, either at home, at work, or both? If so, can you delegate some of your tasks? Can others assist you? Can you say no to new responsibilities? Assess and monitor your daily and weekly responsibilities, and do your best not to overextend yourself.

4. **Learn to relax.** Develop a strategy that helps you relax when you find yourself becoming stressed (better yet, be proactive and practice it daily to prevent stress). Proven stress-reduction strategies include exercise, deep breathing and muscle relaxation techniques, as well as a good laugh (see page 211). Any or all of these options generally provide a positive outlet for stress so that you can stay on track with your weight-loss program.

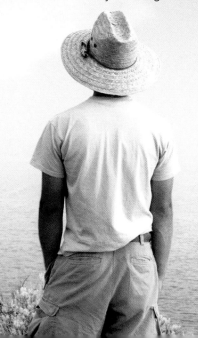

one strategy that you feel is practical and doable.

Locking yourself out of the kitchen and carrying no money with you are two ways to prevent snacking, but they aren't realistic. Taking time over your noon hour to eat a healthy lunch and exercise is more realistic. Retain your other strategies as backups.

5. **Devise a plan to promote this strategy.** How will you go about making sure that you have the time to eat and exercise during the day? One option might be to reserve 30 minutes to an hour every day over the lunch hour for you — a time when nothing else is scheduled.

6. **Identify obstacles.** Look for potential conflicts that might interfere with your strategy and make contingency plans. For example, if you can't find time to exercise, try exercising in the morning before work.

7. **Set a date when you want to achieve your goal — making the changed behavior routine.**

Establish a comfortable pace for change. Depending on what kind of behavior you're trying to change, it may take you only a few days, or it may take you several weeks or months. Jot the date down in your journal. **JOT IT** ▶

8. **When you reach the goal date, evaluate your success.** What worked and what didn't? What would you do differently? If you didn't reach your goal, why not? What got in your way?

9. **Consider what you need to do to maintain this change.** Reaching your goal doesn't mean that now you can stop doing what you've been working so hard at. If you start letting work responsibilities erode your lunch hour, you'll be back to your old habit of skipping lunch and snacking all day. Think about what you need to do to make your healthy behavior permanent.

10. **When ready, select another unhealthy behavior and restart the process.** Use the insight you've gained from previous

behavior-change efforts to help you be successful in your future attempts.

More tips for behavior change

In addition to the strategies you just read about, there are other steps you can take that may help you:

+ **Keep a food diary.** It helps to understand what causes a behavior before you try to change it. One of the best ways to do that is to keep a diary that shows not just what you eat, but what triggers your eating, even when you're not hungry. Use *The Mayo Clinic Diet Journal,* a notebook, or an online journal or app to track what you eat and what prompts you to eat. **JOT IT** ▶

+ **Be mindful.** When you eat, keep your mind focused on the pleasure of what you're doing. Be aware of every bite. To stay focused, you can't be doing anything else — don't read or watch TV, just savor your food. Eating should give you pleasure, not just provide fuel for your body.

+ **Stick to a schedule.** If your diary indicates that you eat many times during the day, having a meal schedule can give you a better sense of control. This doesn't necessarily mean the traditional three meals of breakfast, lunch and dinner.

Create a schedule that's convenient and enables you to eat when you're hungry. Build flexibility into the schedule by defining half-hour or hour time frames for eating rather than setting exact times.

You may find that eating three meals and two snacks works best for you. Or perhaps six mini-meals suit your schedule better. The important thing is to stick with a routine. But don't go more than four or five hours without eating because you could become extremely hungry, causing you to overeat.

+ **Plan ahead.** Try to plan what you're going to eat for the day at least one day in advance. Your decisions will depend, in part, on your daily servings goals. Planning ahead means you'll have the ingredients on hand at mealtimes and can start preparing food without delays. This helps keep you from grabbing a slice of leftover pizza when you arrive home hungry.

Planning ahead also means packing your lunch, snacks or even breakfast to take to work. This saves you from relying on vending machines or fast-food fare and from making impulsive food choices. A good rule of preparedness is always to have something ready that's healthy to munch on, such as low-calorie popcorn, cut-up vegetables or fruit.

+ **Find your eating place.** Designate an appropriate place in the house for eating, preferably at a dining table. Set the table, even if you're eating alone. Make the environment as pleasant as possible, and one without distractions. By eating in one place, you begin to associate that place — and that place only — with eating.

+ **Manage your temptations.** You might trick yourself into believing

Make it realistic and enjoyable

One of the most important steps to successful weight control is to have realistic goals and expectations. If you set your expectations too high or hold yourself to impossible goals, you're setting yourself up for failure.

Start small and take one day at a time. If you understand what's possible in the context of your everyday life and work within those parameters, you're more likely to succeed.

It's also important that you enjoy and find satisfaction in the changes you're making to your lifestyle. Consciously include satisfaction in your goal setting. A study of individuals who successfully managed their weight after completing a medically supervised weight-loss program showed that satisfaction with the amount and quality of daily activities was an important factor in their success. If you don't like what you're doing to lose weight, you won't stick with the program.

As you think about your goals and expectations, look at your results from *Lose It!* Flip through your journal to find what worked and what didn't, and what you enjoyed and what you didn't. Build on that in your long-term goals.

that the bag of chocolate-covered peanuts you tossed into your shopping cart is for a special occasion, but once it's in the house, can you resist having a sample? Do yourself a favor. Don't buy high-calorie foods that tempt you to snack.

+ **'Out of sight, out of mind.'** If you do need to keep tempting foods in the house, store them where you can't see them, especially if your diary reveals that your urge to eat is triggered by visual cues.

+ **Eat from hunger, not emotion.** Food is comforting, and many people reach for food when they try to resolve a problem. Because of this, people tend to forget what real hunger feels like. Don't eat for a few hours and see how you feel.

If what you experience isn't physical hunger, don't try to comfort yourself with food. If you're tired, then rest or meditate. If you're thirsty, drink a glass of water. If you're anxious, take a walk. Stop making eating your all-purpose response to every situation.

When you have an urge to eat, but you're not sure whether you're hungry, wait 15 to 30 minutes and see how you feel. Here's a clue: If you can't decide what you want to eat, chances are you're not very hungry.

+ **Stop when you're full.** No matter what you may have heard from your parents as a child, you don't have to finish all the food on your plate. Even if you served yourself what you considered a reasonable portion, how do you know before you start eating how much food will satisfy your hunger?

Eat slowly, savor every bite, and stop when you're full. If you're not good at sensing when you're full, start with a small portion on your plate, and get a little more if you need to.

+ **Address stress.** Eating is often associated with stress. But eating to ease stress almost always results in overeating. Finding other ways to cope with stress may prevent a lapse and unnecessary weight gain.

Try these ideas to help reduce or manage everyday stress:

▸ Prioritize, plan and pace your activities. Don't try to pack in a lot in a little amount of time.
▸ Get enough sleep to help clear your mind and make you ready for the day.
▸ Get plenty of exercise. During physical activity your body releases specific chemicals (endorphins and enkephalins) that help alleviate stress and anxiety.
▸ Take stretch breaks throughout the day.
▸ Spend time with people who have a positive outlook and sense of humor. Positive vibes rub off!
▸ Organize your work spaces so that you know where things are.
▸ Learn to delegate responsibility.
▸ Don't feel guilty if you're not productive every minute of every day. Take time to relax.
▸ Socialize and spend time with people you enjoy.
▸ Do something good just for yourself or for somebody else.
▸ Take a day off with no set plans.

One step at a time

We tend to be comfortable with our behaviors and habits, even if they're not always enjoyable or beneficial. They're familiar. They give order and stability to our lives.

Although change can be difficult, it's not impossible. Most people underestimate their ability to change. And changing behaviors in many small ways can add up to a big difference in lifestyle.

Here's a common dietary example: Many people have switched from drinking whole milk to skim milk. Maybe they tapered off gradually and changed to 2% milk first, or maybe they switched from one to the other in one bold leap. Either way, they made what they thought was an impossible change. Skim milk probably seemed watered down at first. Now that these people are used to skim, whole milk probably tastes too thick and rich. At first, change may seem difficult, but after it becomes part of your new routine, it seems much easier.

Take a moment to think about other changes you've faced in your life and how you adjusted. The strengths you relied on then may help you now. Use them.

Chapter 19
Burning even more calories

If you want to burn calories, move. If you want to burn even more calories, move more. It's pretty much that simple. Chapter 10 touched on some of the basics of burning calories through increased physical activity. Here, we go into a little more depth.

The cool thing about burning calories is that the possibilities are almost endless. You don't even have to break a sweat.

You can go long — as in duration — with low intensity, mainly moving a lot throughout the day. Or, if a bit of perspiration doesn't turn you off, you can burn a lot of calories with short, high-intensity activity — if you can handle it (see page 215).

A balanced program includes aerobic activities and resistance training to help burn calories, and core stability exercises and stretching to make your activities safe and more effective.

Be flexible in your planning. Create a routine that fits your schedule and interests. Maybe you can walk for an hour on most days and do resistance training for 20 minutes three times a week. Do what works for you.

Once you're in the habit, exercising regularly will feel comfortable. You may look forward to taking a break from other obligations. And remember, you don't have to do your daily exercises all at one time.

Key points

Whether you go with low-intensity physical activity or full-blown exercise, remember these key points:

+ Start with activities that match your current fitness level and gradually build upon them to reach a higher level.
+ When building up, first increase the frequency of your exercise (number of days a week), then as you become more fit, the duration (length of each activity session) and the intensity (how hard you're working).
+ Make sure to pick activities that you enjoy so you'll stick with them.
+ Keep physical fitness in balance with the rest of your life (but make it an important part of that balance).

Schedule time for rest in your routine. Your body needs to recover between exercise sessions. Alternate between low-intensity and higher intensity exercise from day to day.

The following pages give you a little more depth on aerobics, resistance training, core training and stretching.

How to become more active

A simple walking program, such as the example below, may be the best aerobic activity to start with, especially if you haven't been particularly active. Begin with slow, short walks and gradually increase your frequency, time and intensity.

Once you can walk a distance without much strain, you can vary the intensity by walking hills, increasing your pace or swinging your arms more. Also consider including other types of physical activity.

Your overall goals are to move each day, perform aerobic activities most days of the week, and incorporate resistance training and flexibility exercises two to three days a week. Design your program to suit your needs, aiming for about an hour of physical activity each day.

Week	Minutes/day	Comments
1	15	4 days this week
2	20	5 days this week
3	25	Begin 7 days a week
4	30	
5	35	
6	40	Increase intensity
7	45	
8	50	
9	55	
10	60	Increase intensity

Aerobic exercise

Aerobic activities are those that are low enough in intensity that they can be maintained for long periods (30 to 60 minutes) but high enough in intensity that your heart rate and respiration rates will increase, and you may sweat.

Aerobic activities increase your energy expenditure, so you burn more calories. Do them most days of the week.

An aerobic workout should include:

+ **Warm-up phase.** Before your activity, warm up for five to 10 minutes to gradually rev up your cardiovascular system and increase blood flow to your muscles. Try a low-intensity version of your planned activity. If you plan to walk, warm up by walking slowly.

+ **Conditioning.** Perform your planned aerobic activity.

+ **Cool-down phase.** After conditioning, cool down for five to 10 minutes. Stretch your calf muscles, upper thighs, hamstrings, lower back and chest. After-workout stretching improves muscle flexibility and allows your heart rate to return to normal.

Speed calorie burn with higher intensity

If you're interested in burning even more calories, and you're physically capable of stepping up your program, higher intensity exercise may help.

When you exercise, the increase in activity boosts the number of calories you burn, not just during the activity but for a while afterward as well. With low-intensity activities, the afterburn tails off fairly quickly. But with higher intensity activities, the afterburn is longer.

Intervals are one example of a higher intensity activity. They involve repeated bursts of relatively intense activity separated by short recovery periods, such as cycling fairly hard for several minutes, then pedaling casually for a minute or two to recover, and repeating this several times. Intervals can also be part of a walking program, by walking fast for a while, then slower, and repeating.

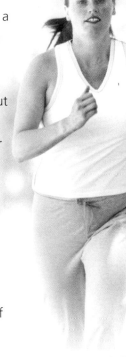

Afterburn also can be extended without the short bursts, simply by increasing the intensity of activity throughout. For example, you could walk more briskly for the duration of your normal walk.

Before increasing the intensity, make sure you're ready — that you've built a good foundation. Remember — frequency first, then duration, then intensity. And check with your doctor if you're uncertain about your health.

WARNING SIGNS: WHEN TO STOP

Moderate activity should cause you to breathe faster and feel like you're working. But if you experience any of these signs or symptoms during exercise, stop immediately and seek medical attention:

+ Chest pain or tightness
+ Dizziness or faintness
+ Pain in an arm or your jaw
+ Severe shortness of breath
+ Excessive fatigue

+ Bursts of very rapid or slow heart rate
+ An irregular heartbeat
+ Severe joint or muscle pain
+ Joint swelling

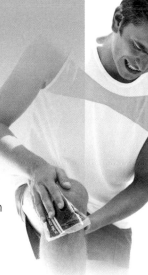

Resistance training

Resistance training, also referred to as strength training or weightlifting, builds the strength and endurance of your muscles. Resistance training reduces body fat and increases lean muscle mass.

Increased lean muscle mass will provide you with a bigger "engine" to burn calories. Because muscle tissue burns more calories than does fat tissue, the more muscle mass you have, the more calories you burn, even at rest.

Resistance training involves working your muscles against some form of resistance. This is typically done with free weights, weight machines or resistance bands.

You can also exercise using the weight of your own body as the resistance, as occurs with exercises such as pushups, lunges and standing squats.

Regardless of the method you choose, begin slowly. If you start with too much resistance or too many repeti-

tions, you may damage muscles and joints. A single set of 12 repetitions (reps) can help you gain strength just as effectively as doing multiple sets.

If you're a healthy adult, begin with a weight you can lift comfortably eight times, and build up to 12 repetitions. The weight should be heavy enough so that the last three to four repetitions are difficult to complete. After you can easily do 12 repetitions, increase the weight by up to 10 percent.

Before each session, take a five- to 10-minute walk to warm up your muscles. You can work your whole body during each session, or you can focus on your upper body during one session and your lower body during the next. To allow time for your muscles to recover, take at least one day off before working the same muscle group again.

If you're new to resistance training, consider working with a certified professional at a fitness center to learn proper technique. Or look for a class offered through a community education program.

Try to do resistance training two to three days a week. Here are some basic guidelines:

+ **Complete all movements slowly and with control.** If you're unable to maintain good form, decrease the weight or number of reps.

+ **Breathe normally and freely.** Exhale as you lift a weight and inhale as you lower it.

+ **Stop if you feel pain.** The intensity level should be somewhat hard, but you shouldn't feel pain.

+ **Change your routine frequently.** Do this to avoid injury and prevent boredom.

+ **Listen to your body.** Mild muscle soreness for a few days after starting resistance training is normal. Sharp pain and sore or swollen joints can mean that you've overdone it.

+ **Stretch your muscles afterward.** Before your workout, simply warm up your muscles.

Core stability

Your core — the area around your trunk and pelvis — is where all movement in your body originates. It's also where your center of gravity is located. A strong core provides a more stable platform for movement and helps you with other physical activities.

When you have good core stability, the muscles in your pelvis, lower back, hips and abdomen work in harmony and provide support to your spine. A weak core can make you susceptible to poor posture, lower back pain and muscle injuries.

Core strengthening requires the regular and proper exercise of your body's core muscles. Abdominal crunches are a form of core exercise. You can have fun doing some core exercises using a fitness ball. Balancing on these oversized, inflated balls requires that you focus on using your core muscles for support.

Do core exercises at least three times a week. Breathe steadily and slowly, and take a break when you need one. For optimal results, get help from a trained professional when you begin — body position and alignment are crucial when performing core-strengthening exercises.

Stretching and flexibility

Most aerobic and resistance training programs cause your muscles to tighten. Stretching can increase flexibility and range of motion, helping you in your day-to-day activities and in the other components of your exercise program. When stretching:

+ **Warm up first.** Stretching muscles when they're cold increases your risk of injury, including pulled muscles. Warm up by walking while gently pumping your arms, or do a favorite exercise at low intensity for five minutes. You want to stretch your muscles after exercise — when your muscles are warm.

+ **Target major muscle groups.** Focus on your calves, thighs, hips, lower back, neck and shoulders. Also stretch muscles and joints that you routinely use at work or play.

+ **Hold each stretch for at least 30 seconds.** It takes time to lengthen tissues safely. Try to hold your stretches for 30 to 60 seconds, if possible. Then repeat the stretch on the other side. For most muscle groups, a single stretch is usually sufficient.

+ **Don't bounce.** Bouncing as you stretch can cause small tears in the muscle. These tears leave scar tissue as the muscle heals, which tightens the muscle even further — making you less flexible and more prone to pain.

+ **Focus on pain-free stretching.** You may feel tension while you're stretching, but it shouldn't hurt. Back off to the point where you don't feel pain, and hold the stretch.

+ **Relax and breathe freely.** Don't hold your breath.

As a general rule, stretch whenever you exercise. If you're particularly tight, you might want to stretch every day or even twice a day.

You might consider signing up for a yoga or tai chi class, which promote flexibility. Plus, it may be easier to stick with a stretching program if you're in a class.

Calories burned in 1 hour

Calorie expenditure for a variety of activities varies widely depending on the type of exercise, intensity level and individual. If you weigh less than 160 pounds, your calories burned would be somewhat less than shown, and if you weigh more than 240 pounds, calories burned would be somewhat more.

Activity (1-hour duration)	WEIGHT OF PERSON AND CALORIES BURNED		
	160 POUNDS (73 kilograms)	200 POUNDS (91 kilograms)	240 POUNDS (109 kilograms)
Aerobics, low-impact	365	455	545
Aerobics, water	402	501	600
Basketball game	584	728	872
Bicycling, < 10 mph, leisure	292	364	436
Bowling	219	273	327
Dancing, ballroom	219	273	327
Elliptical trainer, moderate effort	365	455	545
Golfing, carrying clubs	314	391	469
Hiking	438	546	654
Ice skating	511	637	763
Jogging, 5 mph	606	755	905
Racquetball, casual, general	511	637	763
Resistance (weight) training	365	455	545
Rowing, stationary	438	546	654
Running, 8 mph	861	1,074	1,286
Skiing, cross-country	496	619	741
Skiing, downhill	314	391	469
Softball or baseball	365	455	545
Stair treadmill	657	819	981
Swimming, laps, light or moderate	423	528	632
Tennis, singles	584	728	872
Volleyball	292	364	436
Walking, 2 mph	204	255	305
Walking, 3.5 mph	314	391	469
Yoga, hatha	183	228	273

Adapted from Ainsworth BE, et al., *Medicine and Science in Sports and Exercise*, 2011;43:8.

Chapter 20
I slipped up — what do I do?

OK, so you slipped up and fell off your eating plan. That happens. Everyone experiences challenges sooner or later. It doesn't do any good to get all bent out of shape about it. You can't change the past. What does help is analyzing what happened so you can try to avoid the situation again.

Even with a good plan and the best of intentions, you'll run into obstacles now and then. How you respond to these obstacles can be the difference between success and failure.

Here's a look at some common problems that can cause a lapse in your eating and exercise plans and what you can do about them.

Plateaus

There's no greater reward for your effort than to step on the scale and see that you've lost weight. But what happens when the indicator on the scale doesn't change from week to week, even if you're eating a healthy, low-calorie diet and exercising regularly? Or you see results for the first few weeks, then hit a plateau? Days may go by, occasionally weeks, when your weight remains unchanged.

Before you get discouraged, understand that long-term results don't always show up right away. It's normal to hit plateaus. Some may even be due to your program. For example, exercise builds muscle. Muscle weighs

more than fat. You can have more muscle, less fat, look trimmer but not weigh less. Still, you've made progress that the scale doesn't show.

Above all, when you hit a plateau, don't give up! Appreciate the progress you've made, and keep going. But make sure you're on track with weight-loss basics. Review the strategies in the Action Guide. Or try one of these tips:

+ Review your food and activity records. **JOT IT** ▸ Make sure you haven't loosened the rules, letting yourself get by with larger portions or less exercise.

+ Focus on three- to four-week trends in weight loss instead of daily fluctuations. You may find that, although progress is not evident immediately, you're losing weight.

+ If you've hit a plateau, reassess your program. Is it possible that you've accomplished about as much as you can with the goals you've set? If you're unable to eat less or move more, you may need to adjust your goals.

Lapse and relapse

A lapse occurs when you revert to old behaviors once or twice. It's temporary, common and a sign that you need to get back in control.

A relapse is more serious. After several lapses have occurred in a short span of time, you're at risk of completely reverting back to your old behaviors. When you experience a lapse, you may panic, afraid that you'll undo all your good efforts. You may say, "I guess I just can't do it."

Calm down and take a deep breath. Remember that lapses are normal and can be anticipated. Consider these tips for getting back on track so that a lapse doesn't become a relapse:

+ **Don't let negative thoughts take over.** Remember that mistakes happen and that each day is a chance to start anew.

+ **Identify the problem, then create a list of possible solutions.** Pick a solution to try. If it works, then you've got a plan for preventing another lapse. If it doesn't work, try the next solution and go through the same process until you find one that works.

+ **Get support.** Talk to family, friends or a professional counselor.

+ **Work out your guilt and frustration with exercise.** Take a walk or go for a swim. Keep the exercise upbeat. Don't use exercise as punishment for a lapse.

+ **Recommit to your goals.** Review them and make sure they're still realistic. Makes changes if needed, and consider repeating *Lose It!*

What if you do relapse? Although relapses are disappointing, they can help you learn that your goals may be unrealistic, that certain situations create challenges or that certain strategies don't work.

Above all, realize that reverting to old behaviors doesn't mean all hope is lost. It just means you need to recharge your motivation, recommit to your program and return to healthy behaviors.

Behavior chains

It's happened to everyone. You had a good day — you biked to work, you had fresh fruit for breakfast and you took a 15-minute walk during your lunch break. Then a midafternoon craving sent you sprinting for the vending machine. Three minutes later, you're at your desk with an extra-large candy bar in hand.

What happened? Maybe you were tired, or you didn't eat enough at lunch. Whatever the reason, you let a craving get the best of you. Now you feel guilty and frustrated and you're angry with yourself — feelings that could very well send you back to the vending machine. Where do you go from here?

Imagine this chain of events as a series of separate but interconnected behaviors. To learn how you can prevent a small mistake from becoming a big one, let's separate a behavior chain into discrete parts. By examining each link you'll learn strategies for ways to prevent future lapses from becoming relapses.

Take the example of a woman who feels guilty after eating cookies but continues to eat more. Here's her chain of behavior:

1. Agrees to bring cookies instead of a salad to a friend's potluck dinner
2. Buys the cookies two days beforehand
3. Works late and misses her lunch
4. Arrives home very hungry
5. Thinks, "I'll eat one cookie, then find something to make for dinner."
6. Takes the box of cookies to the den
7. Eats cookies while watching television and reading her mail
8. Eats the cookies rapidly and without awareness
9. Feels guilty and like a failure
10. Eats more
11. Quits her weight-loss program

At every link, she could have done something to break the chain of events. She could have agreed to bring a salad or a dessert she doesn't crave. She could have waited until the day of the party to buy the cookies. She could have prepared an evening meal in advance, so that after missing lunch, her eating wouldn't get out of control

Accentuate the positive

You start your day by stepping on the scale, and as the needle rises, you think, "I'll never be able to lose this extra weight." Maybe you decide to skip your morning walk because "it won't work anyway." At breakfast, you're so down that you top off your cereal with a doughnut and a glass of chocolate milk because, you think to yourself, "I've already blown my diet anyway. What does it matter?"

The scenario isn't uncommon, but it is unhealthy. Negative thoughts and attitudes can sabotage your weight-loss efforts. After all, why eat healthy meals and go to the gym if defeat is certain?

The endless stream of thoughts running through your head every day is called self-talk. Often critical and negative, self-talk can discourage and weaken you to the point of despair.

You think: "I'm too fat." "I don't have any willpower." "The weight is coming off too slowly." "There must be something wrong with me."

On the other end of the spectrum is positive self-talk, which can be a powerful tool for building self-confidence, correcting bad habits, focusing attention, and

when she got home. She could have taken one or two cookies into the den, not the entire box. Finally, she could have told herself that this was a lapse and she shouldn't give up.

Remember this whenever you encounter a behavior chain. Try interrupting the chain at the earliest link. If a midafternoon craving regularly strikes, you can break the chain by keeping a healthy snack in your office desk. If you're always famished when you get home, have a dinner prepared that you just have to heat up or pull out of the refrigerator.

powering your exercise and eating routines. Positive self-talk is motivating and encouraging — the basis for many a successful life change. You're using positive self-talk when you bike up that steep hill, repeating all the while, "I can do it! I can do it!"

With a little practice, you can turn your negative self-talk into positive self-talk. Throughout the day, stop and evaluate what you're thinking. Question thoughts that you feel are upsetting, and then practice turning negative thoughts into positive statements. For instance, instead of saying, "It will never work," say, "I'll give it a try."

Some people find that they need outside help to change their negative thoughts into positive affirmations and to rid themselves of self-defeating attitudes and beliefs.

What's called cognitive behavioral therapy may help you do this. Cognitive behavioral therapy is based on the belief that much of what you are is what you think — that how you feel is a result of how you think about yourself and your life. If you're like many people, you allow your feelings to control your judgment. ("I feel fat and ugly, so I must be fat and ugly!") You also magnify negative aspects of a situation while filtering out positive ones. ("I've lost 5 pounds — but it's only 5 pounds, and I'll probably gain it back.")

With cognitive behavioral therapy, a licensed therapist helps you learn to replace these negative thoughts with more positive, realistic perceptions. Once you've learned new ways to view the events that make up your day, you're better able to cope with them.

You will face temptation, so have a plan to deal with it.

Here are four different approaches to help break a behavior chain. Find one that works for you. If the first isn't successful, try another. Different approaches may work on different days.

ABC approach

Heading off problems before they develop can be effective in changing your behavior. This is sometimes called the ABC method: A stands for antecedent, B for behavior and C for consequence. Most behaviors have a cause or antecedent. And behaviors lead to consequences.

Generally, people are more aware of the consequences of a behavior because these often demand their immediate attention. By addressing antecedents first, you may avert behaviors before they start and thus not have to deal with any consequences.

For example, keeping a tub of ice cream in the freezer (antecedent) may cause you to sneak spoonfuls throughout the day (behavior), ultimately causing you feelings of guilt and disrupting your weight-loss program (consequence).

Using the ABC approach, you decide to keep ice cream out of your house entirely. This addresses the antecedent and helps you stick with your plan.

Distraction approach

Imagine that ever since you were a child, you've enjoyed a bowl of ice cream before going to bed. So now, when you get ready for bed each night, the carton you've hidden in the back of the freezer starts calling your name. Focus on turning your attention away from your craving. For instance, you might read, listen to music, write a letter or switch on the television.

Whatever your solution, the key is to find something that diverts your attention until the craving passes. Cravings are short-lived when your mind is occupied with something else.

Confrontation approach

This approach involves facing the negative consequences of your behavior head-on. For example, if you're craving ice cream, think about the unnecessary calories and fat you'll be consuming.

Think about how tired and sluggish you'll feel afterward. Think about how overeating will impact your health. Remind yourself that this isn't what you want to do with your life.

Give yourself a pat on the back for being able to say no to the craving this time. Yes, you can do it! And you will be able to do it again next time — and most times!

How to stay motivated

Staying motivated can help you avoid lapses and relapses. Motivation comes in many forms, but the best comes from within — your own personal reasons for wanting to lose weight. Use the processes outlined in earlier chapters for identifying your personal motivators. Here are some additional tips:

+ **Set goals.** Write them down and post them where you can see them. Focus on short-term goals and not just on a long-term weight-loss goal.

+ **Keep track of your progress.** Record exercise times, servings of food groups, pounds lost, milestones met and improvements in health. **JOT IT** ▶

+ **Put it in writing.** Make a contract with yourself and post it where you can see it.

+ **Use your support team.** Ask your family and friends to cheer you on, and make time to exercise with them.

+ **Reward yourself.** Every time you reach a goal, reward yourself with something that matters to you.

+ **Recognize success.** As you lose weight and become more active, you'll likely feel better. Pay attention to your body to notice these positive changes.

+ **Practice positive self-statements or affirmations.** Repeat them to yourself daily or type them and post them where you'll see them regularly. An example is, "I'm getting stronger and better every day," or that old standby, "Every day in every way, I'm getting better and better."

+ **Cut yourself some slack.** When it comes to your exercise program, remember that you're not in boot camp. It's OK to take a day off now and then when you need it. The more you make your weight program your own, the less likely you are to rebel against it.

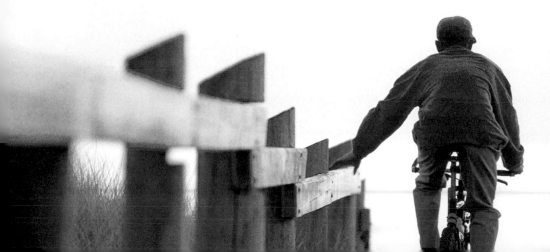

Shaping approach

Shaping encourages you to change your behavior gradually, one step at a time. For instance, instead of cutting ice cream out of your diet entirely, you eat a smaller bowl every night. Then you eliminate one evening snack completely — deciding, for example, to not eat ice cream on Mondays. In time, you'll be able to scale back to a small bowl of ice cream once a week. That's a nice compromise.

In some situations, making gradual changes over time can be less intimidating than making big changes in a single day. As you succeed with step-by-step changes, your confidence will grow and will fuel further successes.

Stress

Stress can sabotage even the best of plans. Everything may be going along well and then something happens that throws a wrench in weight-loss efforts. When stressful situations occur, your natural response may be to abandon your program. You may turn to food for comfort.

This can be the spark for a cycle of unwanted behaviors that puts you at risk of falling back into old habits.

If stress is a problem for you, take steps to deal with it. See Chapter 18 for some tips on coping with stress. If these aren't enough, make an appointment to see a health professional.

If you think your stress may be linked to a mood disorder such as depression or anxiety, see a doctor. In addition to interfering with your plans for losing weight, depression and anxiety require professional help.

Generally, weight loss is easier once treatment for a mood disorder is underway. Be aware that some medications for mood disorders can contribute to weight gain. You might want to discuss possible treatment alternatives with your doctor.

Adjusting your attitude

Maintaining a successful weight program requires more than adjusting your behaviors. The attitudes you have about yourself and about your body

Boosting your self-esteem

Over the years, struggles with your weight may have resulted in some damaging blows to your self-esteem. Some of these may be self-imposed, such as an inability to measure up to your own expectations. Others may come from family, friends, colleagues or even strangers.

It's important to maintain a sense of self-worth. The better you feel about yourself, the better you'll take care of yourself. In addition, a positive self-image has been linked to better health and a stronger immune system.

Many of the steps discussed in this chapter — such as avoiding irrational thoughts, practicing positive thinking and breaking behavior chains — can have a positive effect on your self-esteem. As you learn how to control and positively express your emotions, you'll feel better about yourself and more confident in your abilities — including your ability to lead a healthier life.

On days when your self-esteem could use a little boost, don't be afraid to seek out the support of a friend or family member or do something nice for yourself. You might buy yourself a small gift or treat yourself to a new hairstyle or a massage. Another approach is to think of something that you do well, and then go do it!

When you value yourself, you feel more confident in your ability to meet and solve challenges.

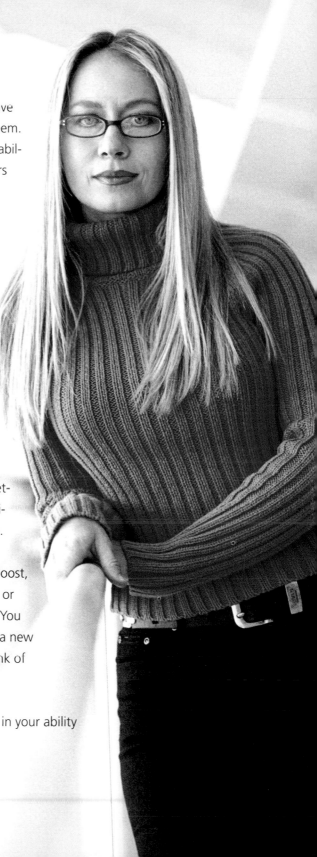

also affect your success. Here are five common problems you may encounter and how to overcome them.

1. Negative self-talk

Self-talk — the internal dialog you have with yourself each day — influences your actions (see page 224). When that self-talk is negative, it can weaken your self-esteem and stall your progress. If you convince yourself you won't lose any more weight, it seems reasonable to say, "Why even try in the first place?"

Remove yourself from this self-defeating behavior by replacing negative self-talk with positive self-talk.

2. Negative attitude

Negative attitudes and beliefs can be as destructive as negative self-talk. For instance, you may believe that you can't go to the gym because people will stare and make fun of your body. Or maybe you credit a special diet for your initial success instead of your own abilities and hard work. Such perceptions can sabotage your ability to lose weight.

Fight back by identifying your negative attitudes. Think of alternative attitudes to counteract them. Consider these examples:

+ **Negative attitude.** "Exercise is painful and boring."

+ **New attitude.** "I like how I feel after being physically active. I'll call a friend to go walking and enjoy the beautiful day."

+ **Negative attitude.** "I'm only losing weight because I'm on this program. Once it's over, I'll regain the weight."

+ **New attitude.** "I'm making this happen by making positive choices. My success will continue even when my program ends because I'm committed to changing my lifestyle for a lifetime."

3. Unrealistic dreams

Sometimes, you may imagine that losing weight will cure all your problems. But you know this is an unrealistic expectation.

Be realistic about what weight loss will do for you. You'll likely have more energy and feel better about yourself, but losing weight doesn't guarantee a better social life or more satisfying job.

Your life may change as you lose weight, but maybe not in the ways that you imagine. Try to counteract unrealistic dreaming with these strategies:

+ **Set realistic expectations.** Recognize your unrealistic dreams, then counter them with more-rational goals.

+ **Set short-term, realistic goals.** Instead of focusing on how happy you'll be after reaching your ultimate weight goal, focus on small, achievable goals toward which you can make progress — ones that you are able to measure daily or weekly. This gives you the opportunity to celebrate successes every week.

+ **Celebrate changed behaviors.** Don't just reward yourself for pounds lost. You're working hard, and there are other achievements to be excited about.

4. Inflexibility

Words such as *always*, *must* and *never* add undue pressure to your program. For instance, you decide that you'll "never eat chocolate again." Or you tell yourself, "I must walk two miles every single day."

Why be so tough on yourself? After all, to *never* or *always* do anything is a lot to ask and may be a path to guilt-ridden lapses.

This kind of thinking doesn't allow you to be flexible. And if you beat yourself up over one momentary slip, it's easy to overlook the progress you're making. Denying yourself something, such as chocolate, may actually fuel a craving.

Once you've broken your rule, you may allow yourself to have chocolate ice cream before dinner or chocolate cake before bed. You feel like a failure.

The sensible approach is to enjoy a treat now and then, but do it in appropriate situations. Have chocolate when you're out to dinner with friends, not when you're alone or feeling sad.

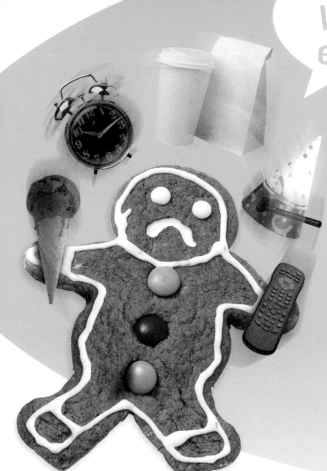

What are your eating triggers?

One way to prevent a recurrence of overeating is to identify situations that cause you trouble. Consider what your eating triggers might be, and plot strategies to overcome them.

Time of day

Are there certain times of the day when you're more susceptible to overeating? Maybe you do well in the mornings and afternoons but have a tough time with food cravings in the evenings. Or perhaps in that lull between lunch and dinner, you get a strong, uncontrollable urge to snack.

Emotions

Food is a common response to a negative mood. Do you find that certain feelings

5. All-or-nothing thinking

All-or-nothing thinking causes you to see a situation as either completely good or completely bad, with no in between.

For instance, you may think, "If I exceed my calorie count today, I'm back to being overweight," or "If I skip the treadmill today, I've blown the program." In short, what you feel is, "If I'm not perfect, I'm a failure."

Few things about weight loss are all or nothing. One setback doesn't mean you're a failure. If you let yourself believe this, you're likely to suffer guilt and depression and take a serious blow to your self-esteem.

cause you to snack mindlessly? Do you tend to eat when you're bored, lonely, depressed, stressed or anxious?

Activities

Do you find that you eat more when doing certain activities? Is reading the newspaper or sitting at the computer without food in hand a problem for you? Do you find yourself constantly snacking while watching television or preparing a meal? Is food how you deal with activities that you don't enjoy, such as paying bills or doing homework?

Social situations

Have you noticed that you eat more when you're around certain people? Maybe it's a good friend who likes to go out to eat or frequently invites you over for coffee and a "little snack." Maybe it's when your partner gets the nibbles, and you eat, too.

Foods

Do you find that you just can't eat some foods in moderation, such as ice cream, chocolate, or chips and salsa? Does the smell of pancakes and sausage or fresh cookies from the oven cause you to completely forget about your eating plan?

Physical factors

Does how you feel cause you to overeat? If you skip breakfast, do hunger pangs cause you to lose control of your eating? When you're fatigued, do you turn to junk food for energy? Do you use food to help distract you from chronic pain?

With all-or-nothing thinking, it's easy to convince yourself that you failed and simply give up.

You can counteract all-or-nothing thinking by taking an approach of moderation. Tell yourself, for instance, that there are no "good" or "bad" foods, and that it's OK to have dessert once in awhile.

Or, instead of calling yourself a failure when you eat more than you planned or you miss an exercise session, remind yourself that slip-ups happen to everyone. With the right attitude, you can overcome them.

Don't forget, tomorrow is a new day and a new opportunity to get back on track. Yes, you can do it!

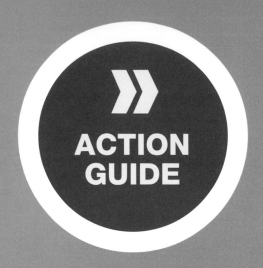

Action Guide to weight-loss barriers

Long-term success with a weight-loss program sometimes follows a bumpy, uneven path. Many obstacles can keep you from achieving a healthier weight.

Learning to identify potential roadblocks and to confront personal temptations are key skills in your weight-loss journey. To make it past the rough spots, you want to have strategies ready to guide your responses as problems arise.

This easy-to-use action guide identifies common weight-loss barriers and practical strategies for overcoming them. If you find a strategy that helps you, include it with your weight-loss program.

The barriers are grouped into three categories: nutrition, physical activity and behaviors. To lose weight — and to maintain that weight loss — it's important that you address all of these components.

❯❯ Nutrition obstacle

I don't have time to make healthy meals.

 Having too little time to cook is a common obstacle to healthy eating. At the same time, preparing your own meals is a key factor in weight control. Even when meal preparations are rushed, it's still possible to follow a healthy diet. Tasty, nutritious meals don't require a lot of cooking time, but they do require that you plan ahead.

❯❯ Strategies

Here are tips to help you eat well on a busy schedule.

+ Plan a week's worth of meals at a time. Make a detailed grocery list to eliminate last-minute trips to the grocery store.

+ Devote time on the weekend to preparing meals for the coming week. Consider making several meals and freezing them in meal-size batches.

+ Remember that healthy meals don't have to be complicated. Serve a fresh salad with fat-free dressing, a whole-grain roll, and a piece of fruit.

+ Keep staple ingredients on hand for making basic meals. For example, you can quickly mix together rice, beans and spices for a Tex-Mex casserole.

+ Have family members help in the kitchen. Split up the tasks to save time.

+ On days when you don't have time to make a healthy meal, stop at a deli or grocery store and purchase a healthy sandwich, soup or prepared entree that's low in calories and low in fat.

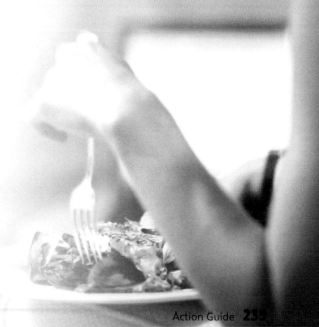

» Nutrition obstacle
I don't like to cook.

Not interested in becoming a gourmet chef? No problem. Many people are reluctant to change their diets because they worry that a healthier eating plan means spending too many hours in the kitchen or struggling with complicated recipes. Healthy eating doesn't require advanced cooking skills, and many healthy meals can be made with minimal time and effort.

» Strategies

If you don't enjoy cooking, here are suggestions to help without a lot of culinary effort.

+ Purchase a cookbook that offers quick and easy healthy meals, or check one out at your local library.

+ Base your meals on fresh fruits and vegetables, none of which takes much preparation or cooking time.

+ Try out a variety of cooking techniques. You might not like baking, but microwaving or grilling may be your thing.

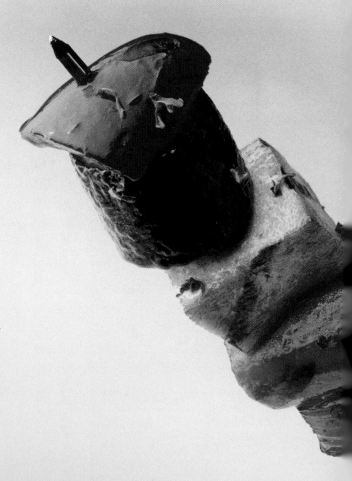

+ Be creative. Use shortcuts such as prepackaged salad greens or raw vegetables, or precooked lean meats.

+ Eat out or order in. It's OK to eat at a restaurant, order in dinner or buy something ready to eat on your way home as long as you choose items that are healthy and you eat moderate portions.

❱❱ Nutrition obstacle
I don't like vegetables and fruits.

Some people find vegetables and fruits boring. Many believe that vegetables and fruits don't have much flavor or that they all taste the same. Not true! Vegetables and fruits are tasty — you just have to know which kinds you prefer and how to prepare them. Much of what you eat is conditioned — over time, you've learned to like it. You still can learn to enjoy new foods, such as vegetables and fruits.

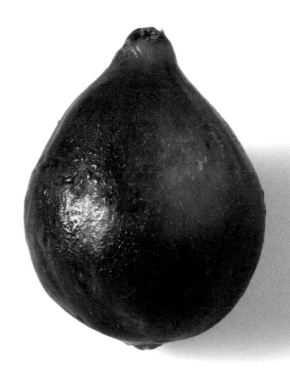

❱❱ Strategies
You can experiment with vegetables and fruits. Here are some suggestions.

+ Keep in mind that you don't need to like all varieties of vegetables and fruits, just some of them.

+ Instead of the familiar apples, grapes and oranges, buy fresh fruits that you haven't tried before. How about kiwis, mangoes, papayas, Bing cherries and apricots?

+ Try using more vegetables and fruits in other foods and recipes: Add vegetables to one of your favorite soups, replace some of the hamburger in casseroles with vegetables, add peppers and onions to your pizza, include fresh fruit with your morning cereal, or mix fruit with yogurt or cottage cheese.

+ Try different ways of preparation. For example, grill pineapple or fruit kebabs. Make fruit smoothies with blueberries and low-fat yogurt.

+ If you don't care for raw vegetables, lightly cook them and see if you prefer the softer texture. Sprinkle them with herbs for flavor.

❱❱ Nutrition obstacle

Healthy foods, such as fresh produce and fish, are expensive. I can't afford them.

Although fresh produce and fish can be expensive, your overall grocery bill may actually be less because you're eating less of other foods, such as red meat, cookies and ice cream. Processed foods can also be costly. Plus, you may find that you're eating more meals at home and fewer in restaurants — this, too, can save money.

❱❱ Strategies

Here are suggestions to prevent the calories in food you buy from adding up at the grocery store.

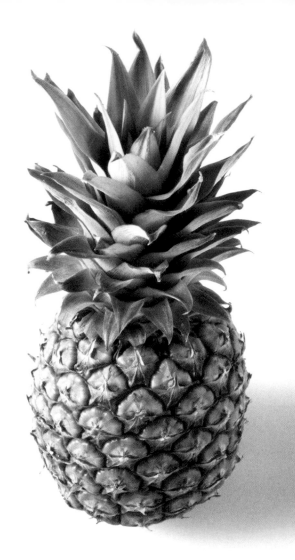

+ A report indicates that, with smart planning, it's possible to obtain your recommended daily servings of fruits and vegetables at a very limited price. Check your options at the grocery store and watch for specials.

+ Buy grains such as oatmeal and brown rice in bulk. Food co-ops are often good at offering foods in bulk.

+ Visit farmers markets for summertime deals. You can usually pick up the freshest produce at the lowest prices.

+ Consider growing some of your own produce. It's not as hard as you think. If you don't have room for a garden, you can grow items such as tomatoes and peppers in outdoor pots.

+ Eat simple meals sometimes. A peanut butter sandwich made with whole-wheat bread or a bowl of soup and a few pieces of fruit don't cost much.

▶ Nutrition obstacle

My family doesn't like to try new foods, and it's too much work to make two different meals.

Family support is important when you're trying to lose weight, but don't let your family stop you from trying something new or exploring different ways of preparing favorite foods. When your family sees you enjoying a meal, your good habits may eventually rub off on them, too. People underestimate their ability to change their tastes. With time, you can learn to enjoy fish as much as steak, or seasoned and roasted vegetables as much as french fries. You may even find you prefer frozen yogurt to ice cream.

▶ Strategies

Here are changes that may help both you and your family enjoy tastes in common and get on the same healthy track.

+ Take it slow. Don't try to overhaul your family's diet overnight. Make a few small changes at a time. Eventually, these small changes add up, and soon you'll all be following a healthier eating plan.

+ Offer a favorite dish that's prepared using a different cooking method. For example, instead of frying pork chops or chicken breasts, bake or grill them.

+ Involve your family in meal planning. Ask family members what they'd like to try that's different and healthy. If they can choose, they might be more willing to experiment.

+ Keep more fruits and vegetables in the house, and keep fruit in a location where it's visible. When looking for a snack, make it easy to grab bananas, pears or grapes.

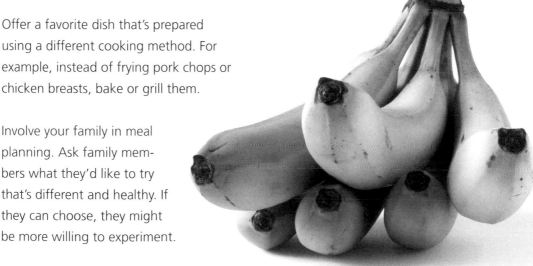

❱❱ Nutrition obstacle
I can't resist certain foods, such as chocolate and candy.

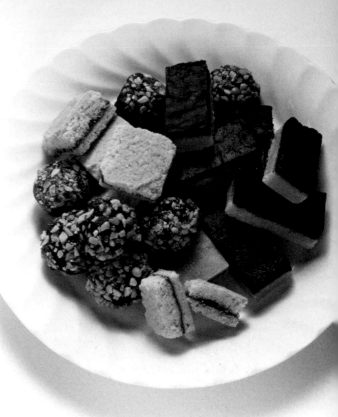

To achieve a goal, you have to be flexible. As you prepare a healthy-eating plan, ask yourself how to fit occasional sweets or junk food into the plan without destroying your overall weight goal. Instead of avoiding these kinds of foods, give yourself permission to eat them on occasion and in moderation. If you try to avoid these foods completely, you'll feel deprived when you can't have them, which leads to disillusionment and to binge eating.

❱❱ Strategies

Here are suggestions that may help you incorporate favorite unhealthy foods into your healthy-eating plan.

+ Plan ahead for the events occurring during the week that put you around sweets and junk food. In appropriate situations — such as going out to dinner with friends — enjoy some of your favorite foods in moderate portions.

+ Know that once you've sampled a favorite food, you may crave more. So it's important to determine in advance how much you'll eat and stick to that portion.

+ Eat healthy foods beforehand so that when it comes time to enjoy a favorite sweet or junk food, you won't be as hungry and will eat less.

+ Don't keep chocolate or junk food at home. If you get an urge to eat such foods, but you have to go out and buy them first, the urge might pass. If you do buy chocolate or junk food, buy it in small amounts, such as single servings.

» Nutrition obstacle
I travel a lot, and I often have to eat at airports, hotels or events.

It can be more difficult to follow a healthy diet when traveling, but it's certainly not impossible. You can find healthy choices when you're away from home. Part of the solution may be your mindset. Avoid rationalizations such as, "I'm traveling, so I'll have to eat whatever is available."

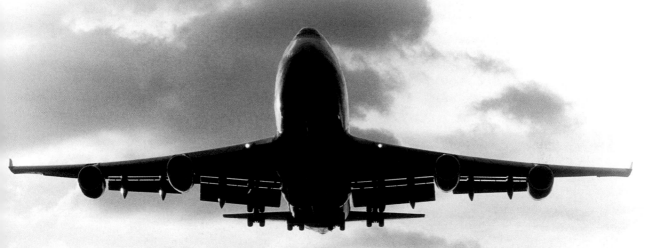

» Strategies
Eating well on the road often requires a little planning before you travel.

+ If you travel by car, pack a cooler with healthy foods, such as sandwiches, yogurt, fruit and raw vegetables.

+ If you travel by plane, pack snacks such as nuts and fruit in your carry-on bag.

+ Ask employees at hotels or conferences about local restaurants that have healthy foods on their menus, or that offer grilled or broiled foods in addition to fried foods. You might also ask if there's a grocery store nearby where you can purchase fruit and easy-to-fix items.

+ At business events, use portion control. Allow yourself small servings of some higher calorie foods so that you don't feel deprived, but eat larger servings of lower calorie foods.

+ Focus your mind on how healthy eating will give you the strength and energy you'll need for your trip.

❯❯ Physical activity obstacle
I don't have time to exercise.

As with mealtimes, too little time for exercise is a common obstacle. With creativity and planning, you can overcome this obstacle. Perhaps you have more time than you realize. For example, the average American watches four hours of television each day. Add to that the time you may spend surfing the web or going on minor errands in the car, and there's bound to be time for physical activity. In most cases, time really isn't the issue; rather, it's a matter of priorities. To become more physically active, it may be that you need to give up another habit.

❯❯ Strategies

If you can't find at least 30 minutes during your day to exercise, look for 10-minute windows. Exercising for 10 minutes three times a day is beneficial, too. Here are strategies you might try.

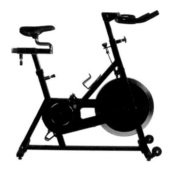

+ Walk for 10 minutes over your lunch hour, or get up a few minutes earlier in the morning and go for a short walk.

+ Take the stairs instead of the elevator, at least for a few floors.

+ Take regular activity breaks. Get up from your desk to stretch and walk around.

+ Instead of always looking for the shortcut from one destination to another, look for opportunities to walk and get more physical activity in your day.

+ Develop a routine that you can do at home. While watching your favorite television program or reading, walk on a treadmill, ride a stationary bicycle or use an elliptical machine.

+ Use the community pool to swim laps or do water workouts.

+ Schedule time with a friend to do physical activities together on a regular basis.

+ While your child is at soccer practice or taking piano lessons, go for a walk or jog.

>> Physical activity obstacle
I'm too tired to exercise.

Maybe that's because you're not exercising enough. Many people find they're less tired once they're involved with a regular exercise program. That's because regular physical activity gives you more energy and because fatigue is more often mental than it is physical. If you're fatigued due to stress, exercise is a great stress reliever.

>> Strategies

To incorporate more physical activity into your day, try these tips.

+ Begin with just five to 10 minutes of activity. Keep in mind that a little activity is better than none. And once you start, chances are you'll keep going for the full 10 minutes — if not longer.

+ Exercise in the morning. This will give you more energy throughout the day.

+ When you get home from work, don't sit down to watch television or use the computer. Instead, put on your walking shoes as soon as you arrive home and go for a walk.

+ Keep motivational messages where you need them to remind you of your goal.

❱❱ Physical activity obstacle
I don't like to exercise.

People who don't like to exercise generally view physical activity as painful or boring. It doesn't have to be either. From among the many forms of physical activity, you're bound to find something enjoyable. You need to experiment. Find something that piques your interest and try it out.

❱❱ Strategies

Here are things you can do to help make exercise more enjoyable.

+ Be mindful. If you're thinking about your to-do list when you're exercising, you may not enjoy exercise. Instead, focus on the moment — the nature around you, your physical movements or your conversation with your exercise partner.

+ Take advantage of introductory classes or exercise videos to learn basic skills and techniques.

+ Mix things up. Don't feel tied to one activity, such as walking. On occasion, try biking or swimming instead. For more ideas on different activities, see Chapters 10 and 19.

+ Focus on the benefits of activity instead of the activity itself. Think of your workout time as time for you. Reflect on your goals, and remind yourself how good it'll feel to achieve them.

+ Listen to music while you exercise. Upbeat music can rev you up and make your workout seem easier. It can also make the time pass more quickly.

+ Think about your typical day. If you interact a lot with people, maybe you'd prefer time to yourself when exercising. In contrast, if you're isolated most of the day, you might prefer being in a class.

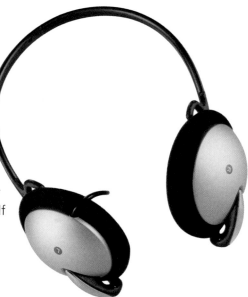

❯❯ Physical activity obstacle
I'm too old to exercise. I might hurt myself.

You're never too old or out of shape to be physically active, and it's never too late to start. Moderate physical activity can help you achieve or maintain a healthy weight. Moderate physical activity can also help delay age-associated illnesses and conditions such as heart disease, high blood pressure, diabetes and bone loss.

❯❯ Strategies

If you haven't been active, it's important to see your doctor before starting exercise, especially if you have some health concerns. Once your doctor gives the OK, here are suggestions for getting started.

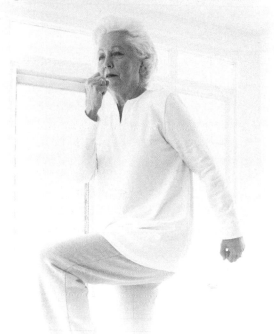

+ Start slowly and give your body a chance to get used to increased activity. Once you're accustomed to the change, gradually increase your activity level.

+ Walking is a good starter exercise. Other options include a stationary bike with no resistance or water exercise.

+ Consider light-resistance exercises, such as the use of elastic bands, for strength training. Studies indicate that even people in their 80s can double their strength at this level of exercise.

+ Do things you enjoy. Activities such as dancing and gardening can provide effective workouts.

+ Stretch. Staying flexible is key to improving or maintaining a full range of motion in your joints and muscles. It's best to do stretching exercises after a brief warm-up period of light activity.

+ Muscle soreness after exercise is common, especially if it's a new activity. Pain during exercise sends a different signal and may require you to stop. For more on exercise red flags, see page 215.

❱❱ Physical activity obstacle

I don't like to exercise when it's cold, rainy or hot.

Choose activities that you can do regardless of the weather, and be flexible with your exercise routine. On days when the weather isn't conducive to your normal outdoor activity, have plans ready for alternate indoor activity. You might also vary your exercise routine according to the seasons.

❱❱ Strategies

Here are some suggestions to consider.

+ Have options for moving your routine indoors. If you bicycle, cycle inside on a stationary bicycle. If you like to walk, walk indoors at a nearby mall or school.

+ Be willing to try something different. Instead of jogging, do indoor aerobics or strength exercises.

+ Swimming in the summer provides a great aerobic workout while also keeping you cool.

+ In colder climates, take advantage of activities such as ice-skating, snowshoeing or cross-country skiing.

+ Check out the local health club. Some don't require that you have a membership but rather allow you to pay per visit.

)) Physical activity obstacle
I worry that other people will think I look funny when I exercise.

Try putting aside such thoughts. Most active people will give you credit for exercising and not make fun of you. Ask yourself which is more important: avoiding feeling possible embarrassment or losing weight. Once you get started, you may find that exercising isn't as embarrassing as you thought it would be.

)) Strategies
If you're concerned about exercising in front of others, consider these suggestions.

+ Most of your self-consciousness will disappear as exercise becomes more routine and you become more confident.

+ Sign up for an exercise class that includes other people trying to lose weight.

+ Buy an exercise video or an exercise machine, such as a stationary bicycle or treadmill, so that you can work out in the privacy of your own home.

+ Exercise early in the morning or late in the evening, when fewer people are around.

+ Ask an exercise professional to demonstrate proper technique and provide information on appropriate exercises so that you can feel confident in your abilities.

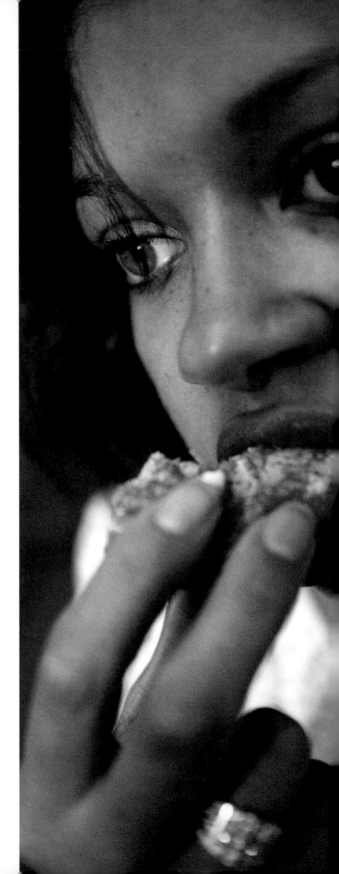

❱❱ Behaviors obstacle
I'm a late-night snacker.

Avoid eating late at night because loading up on calories right before bed only intensifies the challenge of not overeating. There's less chance for you to be active and burn off those calories until the next morning. It's better to eat during the day so that your body has plenty of time to digest the food before you go to bed.

❱❱ Strategies
Here are suggestions if you often find yourself battling the late-night munchies.

+ Make sure you eat three good meals during the day, including a good breakfast. This will help reduce the urge to snack late at night, simply because you won't be so hungry.

+ Don't keep snack foods around the house that may tempt you. If you get late-night munchies, eat fruits, vegetables or other healthy snacks.

+ Find something else to keep you busy in the hours before bedtime, such as listening to music or exercising. Your snacking may be more of a mindless habit than actual hunger.

❯❯ Behaviors obstacle
I have trouble controlling how much I eat.

For many people, a major struggle in reaching a healthy weight is learning how to eat less. Part of the problem is that they don't have a realistic idea of what constitutes a serving. In an era of jumbo meals, supersizing and free refills, overgenerous portions of food and beverages have become the norm. In addition, eating habits that you learned when you were younger — that it's OK to have seconds, that you should clean your plate, that dessert always follows a meal — can be difficult to break. But difficult doesn't mean impossible.

❯❯ Strategies

You can train your body to feel full with less food, in the same way that your body became accustomed to needing more food to feel full. Try these suggestions.

+ Serve meals already dished onto plates instead of placing serving bowls on the table. This requires you to think twice before having a second portion.

+ Try using a smaller plate or bowl to make less food seem like more.

+ Eat slowly. When you eat too fast, your brain doesn't get the signal that you're full until after you've overeaten.

+ Eat the foods that are healthy and low in calories first, before turning your attention to higher calorie foods.

+ Focus on your meal and on your company. Watching television, reading or working while you eat too often leads to mindless eating.

+ Stop eating as soon as you begin to feel full. You don't need to clean your plate.

+ Designate one area of the house for your meals, and only sit there when you eat.

+ If you're still hungry after finishing what's on your plate, nibble on something that's low in calories, such as fresh vegetables, fruit or crackers.

+ Portion sizes in restaurants can be two to three times the amount you need. Request a carry-out container to take the excess home for another meal.

❱❱ Behaviors obstacle
I've tried to lose weight before, but it didn't work. Now, I don't have confidence that it'll work this time.

For many people, losing weight will be one of life's most difficult challenges. Don't be discouraged if you've tried losing weight in the past and you weren't able to — or you lost weight but gained it all back. Many people experiment with several different weight-loss plans before they find an approach that works.

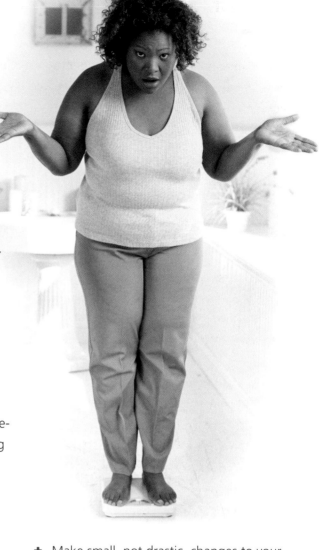

❱❱ Strategies
Following these tips may help you succeed this time around.

+ Think of losing weight as a positive experience, not a negative one. Approaching weight loss with a positive attitude will help you succeed.

+ Set realistic expectations for yourself. Focus on behavioral changes and don't focus too much on weight changes.

+ Use problem-solving techniques. Write down the obstacles that you experienced in previous attempts to lose weight, and come up with strategies for dealing with those obstacles.

+ Make small, not drastic, changes to your lifestyle. Adjustments that are too intense or vigorous can make you uncomfortable and cause you to give up.

+ Accept the fact that you'll have setbacks. Believe in yourself. Instead of giving up entirely, simply start fresh the next day.

➤➤ Behaviors obstacle
I eat when I'm stressed, depressed or bored.

Sometimes your most intense longings for food happen right when you're at your weakest emotional points. Many people turn to food for comfort — be it consciously or unconsciously — when they're dealing with difficult problems or looking for something to distract their minds.

➤➤ Strategies

To help keep food out of your mood, try these suggestions.

+ Try to distract yourself from eating by calling a friend, running an errand or going for a walk. When you can focus your mind on something else, the food cravings quickly go away.

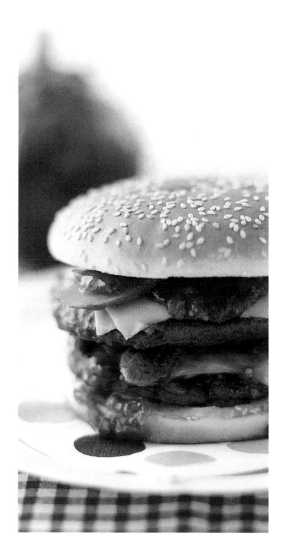

+ Don't keep comfort foods in the house. If you turn to high-fat, high-calorie foods whenever you're upset or depressed, make an effort to get rid of them.

+ Identify your mood. Often the urge to eat can be attributed to a specific mood and not to physical hunger.

+ When you feel down, make an attempt to replace negative thoughts with positive ones. For example, write down all of the positive qualities about yourself and what you plan to achieve by losing weight.

>> Behaviors obstacle

I have a hard time not eating when I'm watching television, a movie or a live sporting event.

There's nothing inherently wrong with eating while watching a show, film or live event, but when you're distracted, you tend to eat mindlessly — which typically translates into eating more than you intended to eat. If you're unable to break this habit, at least make sure you're munching on something low in calories.

>> Strategies

Here are suggestions you might consider.

+ If you're at a theater or stadium, order a small bag of popcorn with no butter and work on it slowly.

+ Eat something healthy before you leave home so that you're not extremely hungry when you arrive.

+ Drink water or a calorie-free beverage instead of having a snack.

+ Try to reduce the amount of time that you spend watching television each day. Studies show that TV watching contributes to increased weight.

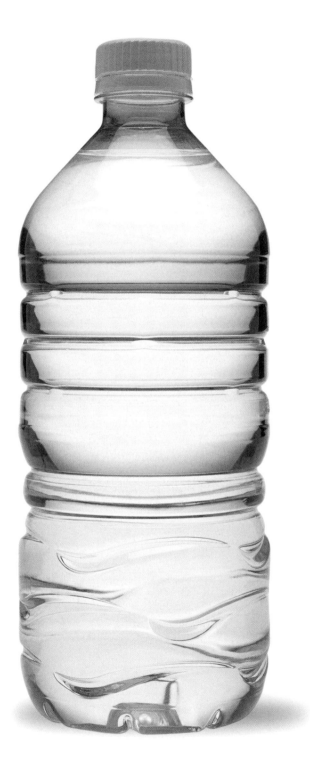

❯❯ Behaviors obstacle
When I go to parties, I can't resist all of the snacks and hors d'oeuvres.

In most social situations where food is involved, the key is to treat yourself to a few of your favorite hors d'oeuvres, in moderation. If you try to resist the food, your craving will only get stronger and harder to control. By following a few simple strategies, you can enjoy yourself without overeating.

❯❯ Strategies

Next time you step up to the hors d'oeuvre table, try these strategies.

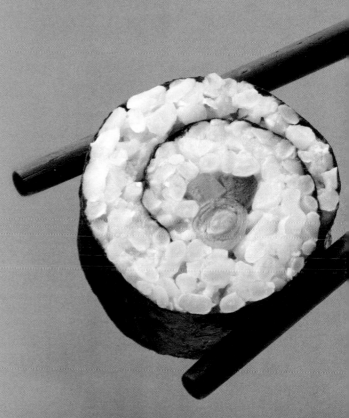

+ Make only one trip and be selective. Decide ahead of time how much you'll eat and choose foods you really want.

+ Treat yourself to only one or two samples of high-calorie or fatty foods. Fill up on vegetables and fruits, if you can.

+ Take only small portions. A taste may be all that you need to satisfy your craving.

+ Nibble. If you eat slowly, you'll likely eat less — but don't nibble all night long.

+ Don't stand next to or sit near the hors d'oeuvre table. As the old saying goes, "Out of sight, out of mind."

+ Eat something healthy before you arrive. If you arrive hungry, you'll be more inclined to overeat.

❱❱ Behaviors obstacle

I get frustrated when I lose just a pound or two after I've tried really hard all week.

Many people long for a secret potion or magic pill that will quickly remove excess weight. Unfortunately, such a remedy doesn't exist. Losing 1 or 2 pounds a week may be frustrating if your expectations are high. But slow and steady is a healthy way to go, and by doing it this way, the weight is much more likely to stay off.

❱❱ Strategies

Follow these tips to keep yourself on track.

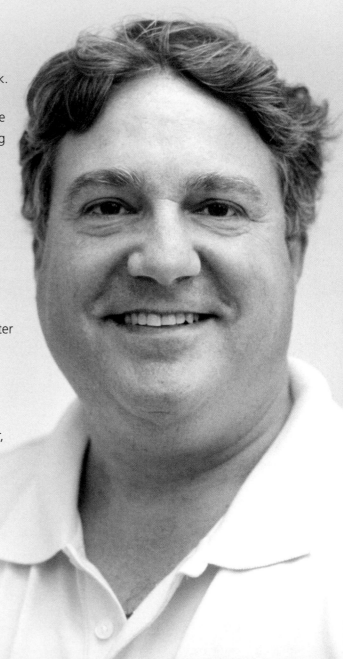

+ Don't focus all of your attention on the bathroom scale. Concentrate on eating better and exercising more.

+ Don't consider yourself to be "on a diet." Try to adopt a positive outlook with the goal of a healthier lifestyle.

+ Make a list of all the benefits of losing weight, such as having more energy, improving your health and feeling better about yourself. Refer to this list if your motivation wanes.

+ Don't use life's ups and downs as an excuse to quit. If stressful events occur, cut yourself some slack if you need to, but stay with the program.

+ Remind yourself that losing 1 to 2 pounds a week equates to about 50 to 100 pounds a year!

❱❱ Behaviors obstacle

I don't like my body image.

How you feel about your body can be central to how you feel about yourself. Many people despair when comparing the way they look to the way they feel they should look. This results in emotional hurt. Having a positive view of your body — no matter how imperfect it may be — is critical to success. To feel good about what you're achieving by losing weight and improving your health, you have to feel good about your body.

❱❱ Strategies

Here are suggestions to help you view your body in a more positive light.

+ Think of your body as a gift. It allows you to live, move, achieve and experience pleasure. If you focus on the good things about your body, it becomes more of a friend and less of an adversary.

+ Don't equate body image with self-esteem. The assumption that how you look is who you are can sabotage your weight goals. Your appearance is only one aspect of your life. You can be a success at many things, regardless of appearance (or how you think you appear). Focus on the things that you're good at.

+ Don't avoid looking at your body. Many people avoid mirrors and windows so that they won't have to look at their reflections. Instead, consider your reflection as a way to measure success.

+ Write a list of positive things about yourself and add to it often. Refer to the list when you need support. In addition, post self-affirming messages ("I'm strong and resilient!") on your bathroom mirror, in your car or at your desk at work.

+ Spend time with people who are positive and supportive of your efforts to lose weight and follow a healthy lifestyle.

+ Get active. When you're physically active you get to know your body better and you feel better about your body. Being spiritually and emotionally active — volunteering in your community, helping your neighbor or getting involved in religious activities — provides purpose and helps you feel better about yourself. This helps improve body image.

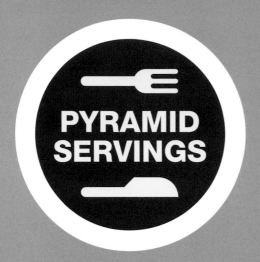

Pyramid servings at a glance

In Chapter 8 you determined your target servings from each of the Mayo Clinic Healthy Weight Pyramid food groups. To achieve those targets, you need to know how much food is in a serving. The lists in this section can help.

Visual guide to servings sizes
See larger chart on page 89.

1 Vegetable serving =
1 baseball

1 Fruit serving =
1 tennis ball

OK, you've realized that not all the foods you eat fit the visual cues from "Quick guide to serving sizes" on page 89. How can you determine pyramid servings? Here's a place to start.

The first part of this section is subdivided according to food groups. It lists individual foods in amounts that equal a single serving. So, by checking the lists, you'll know that if you eat a medium tomato or a half-cup of pasta, it's going to be one serving.

The second part involves "mixed foods," which generally include more than one ingredient (and more than one food group). The separate entries break down servings from the different food groups. So, by checking the lists, you'll know that a peanut butter and jelly sandwich includes carbohydrate, fat and sweet servings.

Important: The serving sizes shown in these lists are "ready to eat" — cooked or raw.

Figuring out your servings

You've just made a small salad topped with olive oil and seasoning. Figuring out your servings begins with your best estimate of the amounts. A good guess is generally good enough.

1 You guess from the size of your bowl that it's filled with about 1 cup of lettuce. In the vegetable listing, you see that 2 cups of lettuce is one serving, so:
+ **1 cup of lettuce in your bowl = ½ vegetable serving**

2 You note that you used about one-half of a carrot, cucumber and tomato in the salad. The list indicates that any of these medium-size vegetables is one serving, so:
+ **½ each of the carrot, cucumber and tomato = 1½ vegetable servings**

3 You learn from the fats listing that 1 teaspoon of olive oil is one serving, which is about what you used. The small amount of seasoning isn't enough to count.

So, the servings breakdown for your salad is:
+ 2 vegetable servings
+ 1 fat serving

1 Carbohydrate serving = 1 hockey puck

1 Protein/Dairy serving = 1 deck of cards or less

1 Fat serving = 1 to 2 dice

Vegetables

Item (25 calories per serving)	One serving is
★ Alfalfa sprouts	1 cup
★ Artichoke bud	½ bud
★ Artichoke hearts	½ cup
★ Arugula	2 cups
★ Asparagus, cooked	½ cup or 6 spears
★ Bamboo shoots	½ cup
★ Bean sprouts	1 cup
Beans, green, canned or frozen	⅔ cup
★ Beans, green, fresh	⅔ cup
★ Beets	½ cup sliced
★ Bell pepper, green, red or yellow	1 cup sliced or 1 medium
★ Broccoli	1 cup florets
★ Brussels sprouts	½ cup or 4 sprouts
★ Cabbage, bok choy, Chinese	2 cups chopped or 1 cup cooked
★ Cabbage, green or red	1 cup chopped or ½ cup cooked
★ Carrots	½ cup baby or 1 medium
★ Cauliflower	1 cup florets (about 8)
★ Celery	1 cup diced or 4 medium stalks
★ Collard greens, cooked	½ cup
★ Cucumber	1 cup sliced or 1 medium
★ Eggplant, cooked	1 cup cubed
★ Jicama (yambean)	½ cup sliced
★ Kale, cooked	⅔ cup

★ **Blue star indicates the best choices.**

FROM THE DIETITIAN

Vegetables are nutritional powerhouses, but they're too often treated as accompaniments or side dishes to the main course. Use their vibrant flavors, colors and textures to expand their role in your diet.

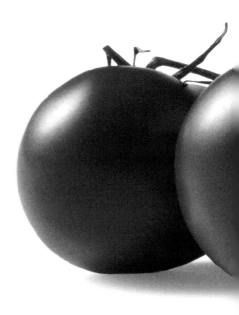

Vegetables

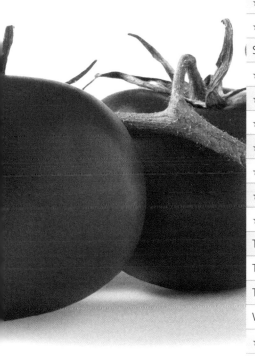

FROM THE DIETITIAN

Looking for corn and potatoes? Many people may consider them vegetables but, due to their nutritional makeup, you'll find them listed with carbohydrates. Green peas are listed with protein and dairy items.

Item (25 calories per serving)	One serving is
★ Leek, cooked	½ cup
★ Lettuce, iceberg	2 cups shredded
★ Lettuce, romaine	2 cups chopped
Marinara and pizza sauce, canned	2 tablespoons
★ Mushrooms	1 cup whole (about 6 medium)
Mushrooms, canned	½ cup
★ Okra	½ cup or 3 pods
★ Onions, sweet, white or red	½ cup sliced
★ Onions, young green (scallions)	¾ cup or 8 shoots
★ Radishes	25 medium
Salsa, vegetable	¼ cup
★ Shallots	3 tablespoons chopped
★ Spinach	2 cups
★ Spinach, cooked	½ cup
★ Squash, summer	¾ cup sliced
★ Tomatillo	½ cup diced or 2 medium
★ Tomato	1 medium
★ Tomato, cherry or grape	1 cup (about 8)
Tomato, stewed, canned	½ cup
Tomato paste, canned	2 tablespoons
Tomato sauce, canned	⅓ cup
Water chestnuts, sliced, canned	¾ cup
★ Zucchini, fresh or cooked	¾ cup

★   **Blue star indicates the best choices.**

Fruits

Item (60 calories per serving)	One serving is
★ Apple	1 small
Apple, dried	⅓ cup
Applesauce, sweetened	⅓ cup
★ Applesauce, unsweetened	½ cup
★ Apricot	4 whole or 8 dried halves
★ Banana	1 small
★ Berries, mixed	¾ cup
★ Blackberries	1 cup
★ Blueberries	¾ cup
★ Breadfruit	¼ cup
★ Cantaloupe (muskmelon)	1 cup cubed or ⅓ small melon
★ Cherries	15 fruits
★ Clementine	2 small
Dates	3 fruits
★ Figs	2 small
Figs, dried	3 small
★ Grapefruit	¾ cup sections or ½ large
★ Grapes, seedless, red or green	1 cup (about 30)
★ Guava	2 fruits or ½ cup
★ Honeydew melon	1 cup cubed
★ Kiwi	1 large
★ Lemon	3 medium
★ Litchi (lychee)	10 fruits or ½ cup
Mandarin orange, canned in juice	¾ cup sections

★   **Blue star indicates the best choices.**

The principle of unlimited fruit servings in *The Mayo Clinic Diet* does not apply to dried varieties such as apples, raisins and dates. That's because when the fruits dry, they shrink — so just a little piece of dried fruit contains a lot of calories! Dried fruit is still healthy, but follow the recommended serving sizes listed in these pages.

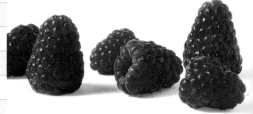

Fruits

Certain foods, such as cranberries and rhubarb, are tart and usually prepared with lots of added sugar before eating. You'll find the serving sizes for these foods listed with sweets. You'll find many juices in the beverage list.

Item (60 calories per serving)	One serving is
★ Mango	½ cup diced
★ Melon balls	1 cup (about 8 balls)
Mixed fruit, dried	3 tablespoons
Mixed fruit cocktail, canned	¾ cup
★ Nectarine	1 fruit
★ Orange	¾ cup sections or 1 medium
★ Papaya	1 cup cubes or ½ medium
★ Peach	¾ cup sections or 1 medium
Peach, canned in juice	½ cup slices
★ Pear	1 small
Pear, canned in juice	½ cup halves
★ Pineapple	½ cup cubed or 2 rings
Pineapple, canned in juice	⅓ cup crushed or 2 rings
★ Plums	2 fruits
★ Pomegranate	½ cup
Prunes	3 fruits
★ Quince	1 fruit (about 3 ounces)
Raisins	2 tablespoons
★ Raspberries	1 cup
★ Star fruit or carambola	2 medium to large
★ Strawberries	1½ cups whole
★ Tangerine	1 large or 2 small
★ Watermelon	1¼ cups cubed or small wedge

★   **Blue star indicates the best choices.**

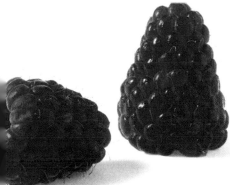

Carbohydrates

Item (70 calories per serving)	One serving is
Animal crackers	6 crackers
Bagel, cinnamon-raisin	½ bagel (3-inch)
★ Bagel, whole-grain	½ bagel (3-inch)
★ Barley, cooked	⅓ cup
Biscuits, plain or buttermilk, from dry mix	1 small
Bread, white or sourdough	1 slice
★ Bread, whole-grain	1 slice
★ Bread, whole-wheat white	1 slice
Breadsticks, crispy	2 sticks (6 to 8 inches)
★ Bulgur, cooked	½ cup
★ Bun or roll, whole-grain	1 small
★ Cereal, cold, bran-type	½ cup
Cereal, cold, flake-type	¾ cup
Cereal, granola, low-fat	¼ cup
★ Cereal, hot (with water), unsweetened	½ cup
Corn, canned or frozen	½ cup
★ Corn, fresh	½ cup
Cornbread, from dry mix	1 ounce
★ Corn on the cob	½ large ear
Couscous, cooked	⅓ cup
Crackers, cheese	14 small
Crackers, matzo, whole-wheat	1 cracker (1 ounce)
Crackers, Melba rounds or Melba toast	½ cup or 6 rounds

★   Blue star indicates the best choices.

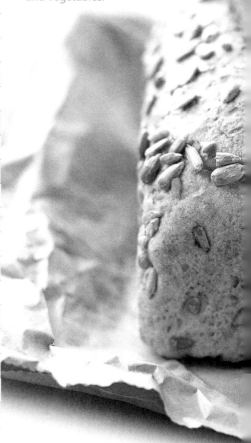

FROM THE DIETITIAN

Carbohydrates are your body's primary fuel supply, and the highest quality fuel comes from whole grains — as well as legumes and fresh fruits and vegetables.

Carbohydrates

High-fiber foods are chewier and take longer to eat, so you consume fewer calories. Fiber also slows how quickly food is digested, which makes you feel full longer.

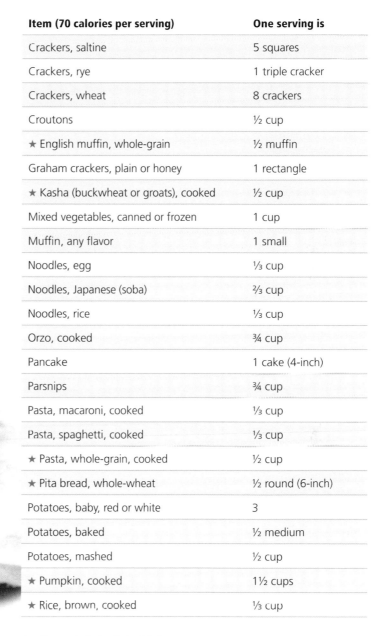

Item (70 calories per serving)	One serving is
Crackers, saltine	5 squares
Crackers, rye	1 triple cracker
Crackers, wheat	8 crackers
Croutons	½ cup
★ English muffin, whole-grain	½ muffin
Graham crackers, plain or honey	1 rectangle
★ Kasha (buckwheat or groats), cooked	½ cup
Mixed vegetables, canned or frozen	1 cup
Muffin, any flavor	1 small
Noodles, egg	⅓ cup
Noodles, Japanese (soba)	⅔ cup
Noodles, rice	⅓ cup
Orzo, cooked	¾ cup
Pancake	1 cake (4-inch)
Parsnips	¾ cup
Pasta, macaroni, cooked	⅓ cup
Pasta, spaghetti, cooked	⅓ cup
★ Pasta, whole-grain, cooked	½ cup
★ Pita bread, whole-wheat	½ round (6-inch)
Potatoes, baby, red or white	3
Potatoes, baked	½ medium
Potatoes, mashed	½ cup
★ Pumpkin, cooked	1½ cups
★ Rice, brown, cooked	⅓ cup

★ **Blue star indicates the best choices.**

Carbohydrates

Item (70 calories per serving)	One serving is
Rice, white, cooked	⅓ cup
Rice, wild, cooked	½ cup
★ Rutabaga, cooked	¾ cup
★ Squash, winter, cooked	1 cup
★ Sweet potatoes, baked	½ large
Taco shell, hard	1 medium shell (5-inch)
Tortilla, corn	1 round (6-inch)
★ Turnips, cooked	⅓ cup
Waffle, frozen	1 waffle (4-inch)

★ **Blue star indicates the best choices.**

FROM THE DIETITIAN

Highly refined carbohydrates have had most of their nutrients stripped away during processing. Although some vitamins and minerals may be added back into products, such as white rice and white flour, they still don't have as many other nutrients as whole grains do.

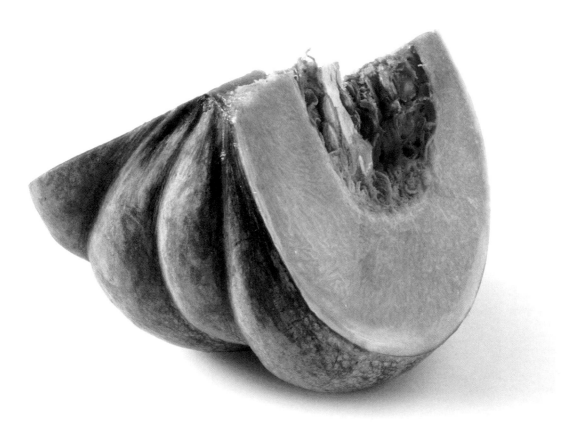

Protein and Dairy

FROM THE DIETITIAN

Proteins are made up of different amino acids, eight of which are called essential because your body can't produce them and they must be obtained via your diet. Common sources of dietary protein include meat, poultry, seafood, eggs, dairy products and legumes.

Item (110 calories per serving)	One serving is
Bacon, Canadian-style	2½ ounces
Beans, baked, canned	½ cup
★ Beans, black	½ cup
★ Beans, chickpeas (garbanzos)	⅓ cup
★ Beans, green soybeans (edamame)	½ cup
★ Beans, kidney	½ cup
★ Beans, navy	¾ cup
Beans, refried, low-fat	½ cup
Beef, ground, regular	2-ounce patty
Beef, ground, 90-95 percent lean	2-ounce patty
Beef, rib-eye steak, trimmed of fat	2 ounces
Beef, sirloin steak, trimmed of fat	2 ounces
Beef, tenderloin, trimmed of fat	2 ounces
Beef jerky	1 ounce
★ Burger, vegetarian	3-ounce patty
Burger crumbles, vegetarian	4 ounces
Cheese, American, fat-free	3 ounces
Cheese, cheddar or colby, low-fat	2 ounces or ½ cup shredded
Cheese, cottage, low-fat	⅔ cup
Cheese, feta	1½ ounces or ¼ cup
Cheese, Gouda	1 ounce
Cheese, mozzarella, part-skim	1½ ounces or ½ cup shredded
Cheese, Muenster	1 ounce
Cheese, Muenster, low-fat	1½ ounces
Cheese, Parmesan	¼ cup grated

★ **Blue star indicates the best choices.**

Protein and Dairy

Item (110 calories per serving)	One serving is
Cheese, ricotta, part-skim	⅓ cup
Cheese, soybean curd	⅓ cup
Cheese, Swiss	1 ounce
Cheese, Swiss, low-fat	2 ounces
Cheese slice, American, processed	1 ounce
Cheese spread, American	1 ounce
★ Chicken breast, boneless, skinless	2½ ounces
Chicken drumstick, skinless	2½ ounces
Chicken giblets, simmered	2½ ounces or ½ cup
★ Clams, fresh or canned	3 ounces (about 10 small)
★ Crab, fresh, imitation or canned	4 ounces
Duck, breast, skinless, trimmed of fat	2½ ounces
Egg, whole	1 large
Egg substitute, liquid	½ cup
★ Egg whites	1 cup (about 6)
★ Fish, Atlantic salmon, grilled or broiled	2 ounces
★ Fish, cod, grilled or broiled	3 ounces
★ Fish, haddock, grilled or broiled	3 ounces
★ Fish, halibut, grilled or broiled	3 ounces
★ Fish, orange roughy, grilled or broiled	3 ounces
Ham	3 ounces
Lamb, lean, ground	2 ounces
Lamb, lean, trimmed of fat	2 ounces
★ Lentils	½ cup
Lobster, boiled	4 ounces

★   Blue star indicates the best choices.

FROM THE DIETITIAN

Milk and milk products are rich in calcium, potassium and protein, and are often fortified with vitamin D. Choose fat-free or low-fat varieties to keep your blood cholesterol levels healthy.

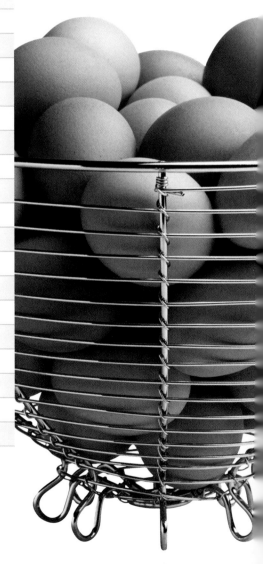

Protein and Dairy

Americans generally consume much more protein than the daily amount recommended by the Food and Drug Administration. Vegetarians may ensure that they're getting enough protein by including lentils, peas, nuts and tofu in their diets.

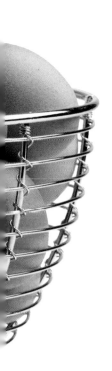

Item (110 calories per serving)	One serving is
Milk, buttermilk, low-fat or reduced-fat	8 ounces or 1 cup
★ Milk, skim or 1%	8 ounces or 1 cup
Mussels	2 ounces
Peas, green, canned	½ cup
Peas, green, fresh or frozen	¾ cup
Pheasant breast, skinless	3 ounces
Pork chops, boneless, trimmed of fat	3 ounces
Pork sausage, smoked	2 small links
Pork tenderloin, roasted, trimmed of fat	3 ounces
★ Scallops	3 ounces
★ Shrimp, fresh or canned	4 ounces
Soy milk, low-fat	8 ounces or 1 cup
Tempeh	2 ounces or ⅓ cup
★ Tofu, firm or silken soft	2 slices (1-inch width)
★ Tuna, fresh or canned in water	3 ounces or ½ cup
Turkey, dark meat, skinless	2 ounces
★ Turkey, white meat, skinless	3 ounces
Turkey breast luncheon meat, fat-free	4 ounces
Turkey meat, ground, cooked	2 ounces
Veal	3 ounces
Venison	3 ounces
★ Yogurt, fat-free, plain, unsweetened or reduced-calorie with fruit	8 ounces or 1 cup
Yogurt, soy, plain, unsweetened	6 ounces or ⅔ cup

★   **Blue star indicates the best choices.**

Fats

Item (45 calories per serving)	One serving is
★ Avocado	⅙ section of fruit
Bacon, pork	1 slice
Bacon, turkey	1 slice
Butter, regular	1 teaspoon
Butter, whipped	1½ teaspoons
Coconut, shredded, sweetened	1½ tablespoons
Cream, heavy	1 tablespoon liquid (4 tablespoons whipped)
Cream cheese, fat-free	3 tablespoons
Cream cheese, regular	1 tablespoon
Creamer, nondairy, flavored	1 tablespoon
Creamer, nondairy, flavored, reduced-fat	1½ tablespoons
Creamer, nondairy, plain	2 tablespoons
Creamer, nondairy, plain, light	2½ tablespoons
Gravy, canned (average of all varieties)	⅓ cup
Guacamole	2 tablespoons
Half-and-half	2 tablespoons
Honey mustard dressing	1½ tablespoons
Margarine, regular or butter-blend	1 teaspoon
Margarine, tub, reduced-fat	1 tablespoon
Margarine, tub, regular	2 teaspoons
Margarine-like spread, light, trans fat-free	1 tablespoon
Margarine-like spread, trans fat-free	2 teaspoons
Mayonnaise, fat-free	4 tablespoons
Mayonnaise, low-calorie	1 tablespoon
Mayonnaise, regular	2 teaspoons

★   Blue star indicates the best choices.

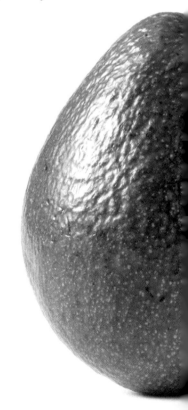

FROM THE DIETITIAN

The fact that there's fat in your diet is not the reason why you may be struggling with your weight. You need to eat some fat because it's vital for a long life and good health. The problem typically is that people eat too much fat, so choose smaller amounts of healthy fats in your diet.

Fats

How you prepare your food can greatly reduce the amount of fat and calories in your diet. Healthy-cooking techniques include baking, braising, grilling, broiling, poaching, roasting, sautéing, steaming and stir-frying.

Item (45 calories per serving)	One serving is
★ Nuts, almonds	4 teaspoons slivered or 7 whole
★ Nuts, Brazil	1 whole
★ Nuts, cashew	4 whole
★ Nuts, hickory	2 whole
★ Nuts, peanuts	8 whole
★ Nuts, pecans	4 halves
★ Nuts, walnuts	4 halves
★ Oil, canola	1 teaspoon
Oil, corn	1 teaspoon
★ Oil, olive	1 teaspoon
Oil, peanut	1 teaspoon
Oil, safflower	1 teaspoon
Olives, black or green	9 large or 12 small
Peanut butter, chunky or smooth	1½ teaspoons
Salad dressing, French, fat-free	2 tablespoons
Salad dressing, French, regular	2 teaspoons
Salad dressing, Italian, fat-free	4 tablespoons
Salad dressing, Italian, regular	1 tablespoon
Salad dressing, ranch, fat-free	3 tablespoons
Salad dressing, ranch, regular	2 teaspoons
Salad dressing (mayonnaise-type), fat-free	3 tablespoons
Salad dressing (mayonnaise-type), regular	2 teaspoons
★ Seeds, flaxseed, ground	1 tablespoon

★ **Blue star indicates the best choices.**

Fats

Item (45 calories per serving)	One serving is
★ Seeds, pumpkin	1 tablespoon
★ Seeds, sesame	1 tablespoon
★ Seeds, sunflower	1 tablespoon
Shortening, vegetable	1 teaspoon
Sour cream, fat-free	4 tablespoons
Sour cream, regular	2 tablespoons
Tartar sauce	1 tablespoon
Tartar sauce, low-fat	2 tablespoons
Whipped topping, nondairy	4 tablespoons

★ Blue star indicates the best choices.

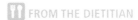

FROM THE DIETITIAN

Monounsaturated fats and polyunsaturated fats — the so-called healthier fats — are found in many vegetable oils, fish, olives and nuts. Saturated fats and trans fats are unhealthy and found in many animal-based foods. All types of fats are calorie dense and should be eaten in moderation.

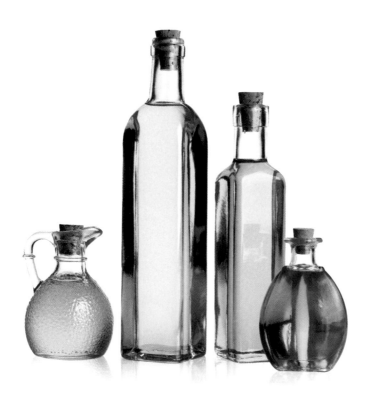

Sweets

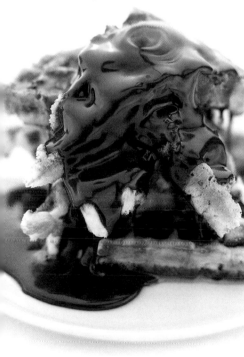

FROM THE DIETITIAN

A craving for sweets is often something you've learned — which means you can also change your taste for sweets by gradually reducing how much sugar you eat and by eating healthier foods.

Item (75 calories per serving)	One serving is
Chocolate chips, semisweet	4 tablespoons
Cranberry sauce, canned, sweetened	3 tablespoons
Frosting, chocolate, ready-to-eat	1 tablespoon
Fruit butter, apple	2½ tablespoons
Gelatin dessert	½ cup
Hard candy (butterscotch, lemon drops, peppermint)	4 pieces
Honey	1 tablespoon
Jellies, jams and preserves	1½ tablespoons
Jellies, jams and preserves, reduced-sugar	4 tablespoons
Jelly beans	20 small or 8 large
Molasses	1½ tablespoons
Rhubarb, cooked and sweetened	¼ cup
Sugar, brown (unpacked)	2 tablespoons
Sugar, granulated, white	4 teaspoons
Sugar, powdered	2 tablespoons
Syrup, light corn	1 tablespoon
Syrup, maple	1½ tablespoons
Topping, butterscotch or caramel	1½ tablespoons
Topping, chocolate syrup	1½ tablespoons
Topping, strawberry	1½ tablespoons

Breakfast

Item	Amount	V	F	C	PD	Ft	S
					Food group servings		
Bacon, Canadian-style	2½ ounces				1		
Bacon, fried	1 strip					1	
Bagel, whole-grain	½ bagel (3-inch)			1			
Bagel with egg and cheese	1 sandwich			3	2	1	
Banana	1 small		1				
Biscuit with egg	1 biscuit			2	1	3	
Biscuit with egg and meat	1 biscuit			2	2	2	
Bread, whole-grain	1 slice			1			
Bread, whole-wheat white	1 slice			1			
Cereal, cold, bran flakes	½ cup			1			
Cereal, cold, flake-type with dried fruit, nuts	⅓ cup			1			
Cereal, cold, shredded wheat, sweetened	¾ cup			1			1
Croissant, plain	1 medium croissant			2		2	
Croissant with egg and cheese	1 croissant			2	1	2	
Croissant with egg, cheese and bacon	1 croissant			2	1.5	3	
Doughnut, cake (plain)	1 (3¼-inch dia.)			0.5		3	0.5
Doughnut, raised (glazed)	1 (3¾-inch dia.)			1		2	1
Egg, omelet, western	1 large egg	1			1		
Egg, scrambled	1 large egg				1		
English muffin, whole-grain	½ muffin			1			
English muffin with egg, cheese and Canadian bacon	1 muffin			2	2	1	
French toast	1 slice			1	0.5	1	
French toast sticks	5 sticks			2	1	1	1

V Vegetables	**C** Carbohydrates	**Ft** Fats
F Fruits	**PD** Protein/Dairy	**S** Sweets

Breakfast

Item	Amount	V	F	C	PD	Ft	S
				Food group servings			
Granola, home-prepared	¼ cup			1		2	
Granola, low-fat	¼ cup			1			
Grapefruit	¾ cup sections or ½ large		1				
Hash brown potatoes	½ cup			1.5			
Melon balls	1 cup (8 balls)		1				
Muffin, blueberry (made with low-fat milk)	1 (2 ounces)			1		1	0.5
Muffin, cranberry-orange	1 large (4 ounces)	0.5		2		4	1
Oatmeal, instant, plain (made with water)	1 packet			1.5			
Oatmeal, instant, sweetened (made with water)	1 packet			1			1
Pancake with berries, syrup and trans-free margarine	1 pancake		1	1		1	1
Pastry, cinnamon Danish	1 (4-inch dia.)			1		3	1
Pastry, cinnamon roll with frosting	1 (2-inch dia.)					1	1
Pastry, toaster-type	1 item			1		2	1
Prunes	3 fruits		1				
Quiche with broccoli and Cheddar cheese	6 ounces	1		0.5	2	4	
Scone with fruit (unfrosted)	1 (4 ounces)			2		4	2
Strawberries	1½ cups whole		1				
Waffle, plain, from recipe	1 (4-inch dia.)			1		1	
Yogurt, plain, low-fat, low-calorie sweetener	1 cup (8 ounces)				1		
Yogurt with fruit, low-fat, low-calorie sweetener	1 cup (8 ounces)				1		

V Vegetables C Carbohydrates Ft Fats
F Fruits PD Protein/Dairy S Sweets

Sandwich

Item	Amount	Food group servings					
		V	**F**	**C**	**PD**	**Ft**	**S**
Bacon, lettuce and tomato	1 sandwich	1		2		4	
Cheeseburger, single patty with condiments	1 sandwich			3	2	2	
Chicken, grilled	1 sandwich			2	1		
Chicken cordon bleu, restaurant-prepared	1 sandwich			3	2.5	2	
Chicken fillet, grilled, with mayonnaise	1 sandwich			3	2	2	
Chicken wrap with cranberry sauce	1 wrap			1	1		1
Fish, with tartar sauce	1 sandwich			3	1.5	1	
French dip, restaurant-prepared	1 sandwich			4	2	1	
Ham and cheese, hot	1 sandwich			2	1.5	1	
Ham and cheese, stuffed pocket, microwave	1 sandwich			3	3	3	
Hamburger, California (vegetables, mayonnaise)	1 sandwich	1		2	2	1	
Hamburger, single patty with condiments	1 sandwich			2	1	1	
Hot dog (frankfurter), beef	1½-ounce dog			2	1	1	
Peanut butter and jelly	1 sandwich			2		2	1
Roast beef, plain, restaurant-prepared	1 regular			2	1.5	1	
Steak	1 sandwich			2	2		
Submarine with cold cuts and veggies	about 6 inches	1		3	1.5	1	
Submarine with tuna salad and veggies	about 6 inches	1		3	2	3	
Tuna salad pita	1 sandwich			1	1	1	
Turkey (vegetables, mayonnaise)	1 sandwich	1		2	1	1	
Turkey with ranch, bacon and veggies, restaurant-prepared	1 sandwich	3		4	3	3	
Turkey wrap, smoked	1 wrap			1	1	1	

V Vegetables   **C** Carbohydrates   **Ft** Fats
F Fruits   **PD** Protein/Dairy   **S** Sweets

Salad and Soup

Item	Amount	V	F	C	PD	Ft	S
Salad							
Caesar salad with grilled chicken	11 ounces	3			1	1	
Coleslaw, home-prepared	1 cup	2				1	
Potato salad, home-prepared	1 cup	1		2		4	
Spinach salad with fruit	2 cups	2	1			1	
Taco salad (fast food)	1½ cups	1		1	1	2	
Tossed salad with cheese and egg, no dressing	2 cups	2			1.5		
Tossed salad with pasta and seafood, no dressing	1½ cups	2		1	2	1	
Tossed salad with turkey, ham and cheese, no dressing	1½ cups	2			2		
Soup or stew							
Bean with pork, canned (made with water)	1 cup				1	1	
Beef stew, canned	1 cup	2		0.5	1	1	
Broccoli, cream of, canned (made with low-fat milk)	1 cup	1			1		
Chicken noodle, canned (broth-based)	1 cup			1			
Chili con carne, with beans	1 cup	1			2		
Clam chowder, New England, canned	1 cup				1.5		
Hot and sour	1 cup			0.5	0.5		
Miso (from 1 tablespoon of miso)	1 cup				0.5		
Mushroom, cream of, canned (made with water)	1 cup				1		
Split pea with ham, canned (made with water)	1 cup				2		
Tomato or tomato-based, canned (made with water)	1 cup			1			
Vegetable or vegetable beef, canned (broth-based)	1 cup	1			1	0.5	

Food group servings

V	Vegetables	C	Carbohydrates	Ft	Fats
F	Fruits	PD	Protein/Dairy	S	Sweets

Main Course

Item	Amount	V	F	C	PD	Ft	S
					Food group servings		
Beef, round roast	2 ounces				1		
Beef, sirloin steak, trimmed of fat	2 ounces				1		
Burrito, beef, beans and cheese	1 burrito			1	2	1	
Burrito, chicken supreme with veggies	1 burrito	1		2	1.5	3	
Chicken, dark meat, fried (fast food)	2 pieces			1	2.5	2	
Chicken, white meat, fried (fast food)	2 pieces			1	3	2	
Chicken breast or drumstick, grilled	2½ ounces				1		
Chicken patty, breaded and fried (fast food)	3-ounce patty			1	1	2	
Chicken stir-fry with veggies	1 entree	3		1	1		
Crab cake, breaded and fried	3-ounce cake			0.5	1	2	
Fajitas, beef, pork or chicken with veggies	2 fajitas	2		2	1	1	
Fish, cod, haddock or halibut, grilled or broiled	3-ounce fillet				1		
Fish fillet, breaded and fried	3-ounce fillet			1	1	1	
Fish sticks, breaded and fried	3 sticks			1	1	1	
Kebabs, beef with veggies	1 skewer	2			2		
Kebabs, chicken with veggies	1 skewer	2			1		
Kielbasa, Polish, smoked	3 ounces				1	2	
Lasagna with meat	2½-x-4-inch piece	2		1	1.5	1	
Macaroni and cheese, from mix	1 cup			2	2	1	
Meatballs, Swedish with cream or white sauce	1 cup (about 5 meatballs)			1	2	2	
Meatloaf, lean ground beef	3-ounce slice	1			1	1	
Pasta primavera	1 entree	2		2	1	1	

V Vegetables	**C** Carbohydrates	**Ft** Fats	
F Fruits	**PD** Protein/Dairy	**S** Sweets	

Main Course

Item	Amount	V	F	C	PD	Ft	S
					Food group servings		
Pizza, cheese, regular crust	⅛ of 14-inch	1		1	1	1	
Pizza, cheese, regular crust, frozen	⅓ of 12-inch	2		2	1	2	
Pizza, pepperoni, regular crust	⅛ of 14-inch	1		1.5	1	1	
Pizza, pepperoni, regular crust, frozen	⅓ of 12-inch	2		2	1.5	2	
Pizza, pepperoni, thick crust	⅛ of 14-inch	1		2	1	1	
Pork chops, boneless, trimmed of fat	3 ounces				1		
Pork ribs, country-style, lean	2½ ounces				1	2	
Pork tenderloin, roasted, trimmed of fat	3 ounces				1		
Potpie, beef, frozen	1 pie (9 ounces)	2		2	1	3	
Potpie, chicken or turkey, frozen	1 pie (9 ounces)	2		2	1	3	
Shrimp, breaded and fried	4 ounces			1	1	2	
Skillet meal, "helper," with lean ground beef, chicken or tuna and veggies	1 cup	1		1	1.5	1	
Spaghetti with meatballs and tomato sauce, canned	1 cup	2		2	0.5	1	
Spaghetti with marinara sauce	1 cup	2		2		1	
Taco, beef or chicken, hard shell with lettuece and tomato	1 taco	1		1	0.5	1	
Taco, beef, soft shell with lettuce and tomato	1 taco	1		1	0.5	1	
Tortellini with cheese filling	¾ cup			2	2		

V Vegetables	**C** Carbohydrates	**Ft** Fats
F Fruits	**PD** Protein/Dairy	**S** Sweets

Side Dish

Item	Amount	V	F	C	PD	Ft	S
		Food group servings					
Beans, baked, with pork, franks or beef, canned	1 cup			1	2	1	
Biscuit (fast food)	1 large			2		2	
Bread, garlic	1 slice			1		1	
Breadstick, soft (fast food)	1 stick			1		1	
Buffalo wings	4 pieces				1	2	
Chicken tenders	4 pieces			1	1	1	
Chow mein noodles	⅓ cup			0.5	1		
Crescent roll, from refrigerated dough	1 roll			1		1	
Egg rolls, vegetable, chicken or pork	3-ounce roll	1		1	0.5		
French fries	1 small serving			2		2	
Hummus, home-prepared	4 tablespoons				1		
Mozzarella sticks, deep-fried (fast food)	4 sticks			1	2	3	
Onion rings, breaded (fast food)	8-9 rings	2		1.5		3	
Potato, baked, with cheese and broccoli (fast food)	1 potato	1		3	1	2	
Potato, mashed, with gravy	about ½ cup			1.5		1	
Potatoes, au gratin, with trans-free margarine	½ cup			1	0.5	1	
Potatoes, scalloped, with trans-free margarine	½ cup			1		0.5	
Salsa	¼ cup	1					
Tortilla, flour	1 round (6-inch)			1		0.5	

V Vegetables
F Fruits
C Carbohydrates
PD Protein/Dairy
Ft Fats
S Sweets

Snack

Item	Amount	V	F	C	PD	Ft	S
Bread, banana	1 slice		0.5	1		1	1
Cereal bar, granola-type or fruit-filled	1 bar			1			1
Cheese puff or twist	1 ounce			1		2	
Cereal-based snack mix	½ cup			1		1	
Cracker, sandwich, with peanut butter filling	6 crackers			1.5		2	
Fruit leather pieces	1 pack (¾ ounce)		1				
Popcorn, microwave, buttered	3 cups			1		2	
Popcorn, plain, air-popped	3 cups			1			
Popcorn, plain, oil-popped	3 cups			1		2	
Potato chips, regular	1 ounce			1		2	
Potato chips, baked	1 ounce			1		1	
Pretzel sticks, small	about 30			1			
Pretzel twists	about 3			1			
Rice cakes, most types	2 cakes			1			
Soybeans, dry roasted	2 tablespoons				1		
Strawberry smoothie	1 smoothie		1		1		
Tortilla chips or corn chips, baked	1 ounce			1		1	
Tortilla chips or corn chips, regular	1 ounce			1		2	
Trail mix, with chocolate chips, nuts and seeds	½ cup					5	2
Yogurt, fat-free, plain, unsweetened or reduced-calorie with fruit	1 cup (8 ounces)				1		

Food group servings

V Vegetables	**C** Carbohydrates	**Ft** Fats
F Fruits	**PD** Protein/Dairy	**S** Sweets

Dessert

Item	Amount	Food group servings					
		V	**F**	**C**	**PD**	**Ft**	**S**
Bar, brownie	3-inch square			1		2	1
Bar, lemon	1½-ounce bar					1	1.5
Cake, angel food	1/12 of 12-ounce cake						1
Cake, chocolate, no frosting	1/12 of 9-inch dia. cake			1		3	2
Cake, cinnamon, with crumb topping	1/8 of 8-x-6-inch cake			1		1	1
Cake, gingerbread	1/9 of 8-x-8-inch cake			1		3	1
Cake, pound, fat-free	1-ounce slice						1
Cake, white, no frosting	1/12 of 9-inch dia. cake			1.5		2	1
Chocolate bar, dark	1 ounce					2	1
Chocolate bar, milk	1 bar (1½ ounces)					2	1.5
Cookie, chocolate chip	2 medium					1	0.5
Cookie, chocolate sandwich with cream filling	2 standard					1	1
Cookie, fig bar	2 standard		0.5			1	0.5
Cookie, gingersnap	3 medium						1
Cookie, oatmeal raisin, peanut butter or sugar	1 3-inch dia.						1
Custard	½ cup				0.5		1
Ice cream, light (most flavors)	½ cup					1	1
Ice cream, regular (most flavors)	½ cup					2	0.5
Ice cream, soft serve, vanilla, light	½ cup					1	1

V Vegetables	**C** Carbohydrates	**Ft** Fats	
F Fruits	**PD** Protein/Dairy	**S** Sweets	

Dessert

Item	Amount	Food group servings					
		V	F	C	PD	Ft	S
Juice bar, frozen	1 bar (3 ounces)		1				
Pudding, instant, sugar-sweetened, 2% milk	½ cup				0.5	0.5	1
Pudding, tapioca, sugar-sweetened, 2% milk	½ cup				0.5	0.5	1
Shake, vanilla or chocolate (fast food)	12 fluid ounces				2		2
Sherbet (sorbet)	⅓ cup						1
Pie, chocolate cream, commercially prepared	⅛ of 9-inch dia. pie			1	1	4	1
Pie, fruit (apple, blueberry or cherry), from recipe	⅛ of 9-inch dia. pie		1	1		4	1
Pie, lemon meringue, commercially prepared	⅙ of 8-inch dia. pie		0.5	0.5		2	2
Pie, pecan	⅛ of 9-inch dia. pie			1	1	4	2
Pie, pumpkin	⅛ of 9-inch dia. pie	1		1		3	1
Yogurt, frozen, fat-free	½ cup				0.5		1

V Vegetables	**C** Carbohydrates	**Ft** Fats	
F Fruits	**PD** Protein/Dairy	**S** Sweets	

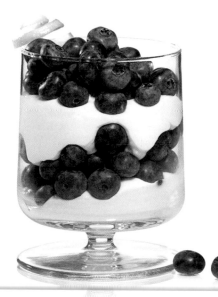

Beverage

Item	Amount	V	F	C	PD	Ft	S
Food group servings							
Alcohol							
Beer, light	12 fluid ounces						1.5
Beer, regular	12 fluid ounces						2
Distilled spirits (gin, rum, vodka, whiskey)	1 fluid ounce						1
Wine, red or white	5 fluid ounces						1.5
Coffee or tea drinks							
Caffé latte or caffé mocha, skim	12 fluid ounces				1		
Cappuccino	12 fluid ounces				0.5		
Chai tea, with skim milk	12 fluid ounces				1		1
Coffee, brewed or instant	8 fluid ounces			calorie-free beverage			
Tea, iced, commercially sweetened	12 fluid ounces						2
Tea, regular or herbal, brewed or instant	8 fluid ounces			calorie-free beverage			
Dairy or cocoa drinks							
Chocolate-flavored mix, made with low-fat milk	8 fluid ounces				1		1
Chocolate milk, made with skim or 1% milk	8 fluid ounces				1		0.5
Cocoa, hot, made with water	6 fluid ounces				0.5		0.5
Milk, 2% or whole	8 fluid ounces				1	1	
Fruit-flavored drinks							
Fruit punch, from powder	8 fluid ounces						1.5
Lemonade, from sweetened concentrate	8 fluid ounces		1				0.5
Orange breakfast drink, ready-to-serve	8 fluid ounces						1.5

V Vegetables   C Carbohydrates   Ft Fats
F Fruits   PD Protein/Dairy   S Sweets

Beverage

Item	Amount	V	F	C	PD	Ft	S
Food group servings							
Juices							
Cranberry, sweetened	4 fluid ounces		1				1.5
Orange, grapefruit or pineapple, unsweetened	4 fluid ounces		1				
Tomato or vegetable	4 fluid ounces	1					
Soft drinks							
Club soda	12 fluid ounces	calorie-free beverage					
Cola, lemon-lime or root beer, regular	12 fluid ounces						2
Cream soda, regular	12 fluid ounces						2.5
Diet soda, any flavor	12 fluid ounces	calorie-free beverage					
Ginger ale, regular	12 fluid ounces						1.5
Sports drink							
Fruit-flavored, ready-to-drink, low-calorie	12 fluid ounces						0.5
Fruit-flavored, ready-to-drink, regular	12 fluid ounces						1
Adding calories to your coffee and tea							
Cream, heavy	1 tablespoon					1	
Creamer, nondairy, flavored	1 tablespoon					1	
Creamer, nondairy, plain	2 tablespoons					1	
Creamer, nondairy, plain, light	2½ tablespoons					1	
Half-and-half	2 tablespoons					1	
Sugar	2 teaspoons						0.5

V **Vegetables** C **Carbohydrates** Ft **Fats**
F **Fruits** PD **Protein/Dairy** S **Sweets**

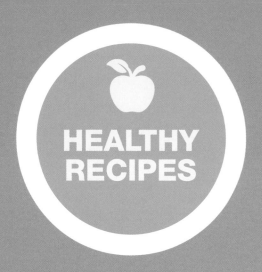

HEALTHY RECIPES

Recipes for weight loss

Can you lose weight and eat well at the same time? Of course! The menu decisions you make each day should be based on a variety of foods and kitchen techniques that can help keep you healthy. The recipes that follow show how easy and enjoyable eating well can be.

Blueberry Muffins

✚ **SERVES 12**

¾ c. all-purpose flour

½ c. whole-wheat flour

¼ c. ground flaxseed

½ tbsp. baking powder

¼ tsp. baking soda

1 tsp. salt

3 tbsp. unsalted butter

½ c. sugar

1 tsp. pure vanilla extract

1 egg

½ c. plain fat-free yogurt

1 c. fresh blueberries

1. Heat the oven to 350 F.
2. Lightly coat muffin tin with cooking spray.
3. Combine flours, seeds, baking powder, baking soda and salt in a bowl; set aside.
4. Using a mixer, combine unsalted butter and sugar until creamy.
5. Add the vanilla and egg.
6. Add the dry mixture, alternating with the yogurt; mix until combined.
7. Fold in the blueberries.
8. Fill each muffin cup with ¼ cup of batter.
9. Bake for 15 minutes.

PYRAMID SERVINGS:

C	Carbohydrates	1
Ft	Fats	1
S	Sweets	0.5

PER SERVING (1 MUFFIN):

Calories	134
Protein	3 g
Carbohydrate	21 g
Total fat	4.5 g
Cholesterol	23 mg
Sodium	231 mg
Fiber	1.5 g

CHEF'S NOTES:

Other fruit can be used instead of the blueberries, such as cranberries, raspberries and chopped apples. You can freeze the muffins for later use.

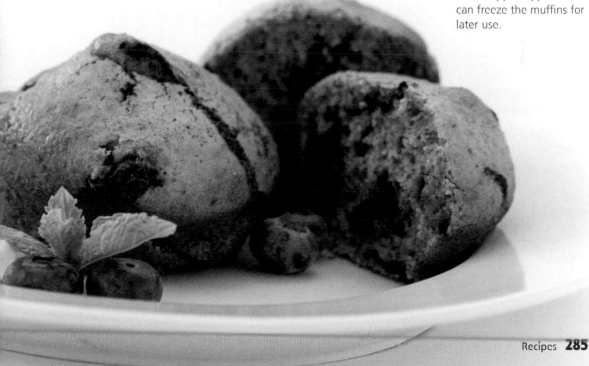

Green Smoothie

+ SERVES 4

1 banana

½ c. strawberries

½ c. blackberries or
blueberries

4 tbsp. lemon juice (or juice
from 1 fresh lemon)

2 c. fresh baby spinach

1 tbsp. fresh mint

1 c. ice

1. Place all ingredients in a blender
   or juicer and puree.
2. Serve or refrigerate.

PYRAMID SERVINGS:

F	Fruits	1

PER SERVING (6 OUNCES):

Calories	50
Protein	1 g
Carbohydrate	12 g
Total fat	0 g
Cholesterol	0 mg
Sodium	14 mg
Fiber	2 g

CHEF'S NOTES:

You can substitute other berries, if you prefer. This drink is an excellent source of vitamins A and C.

Sun-dried Tomato Basil Frittata

✦ SERVES 6

¼ tsp. olive oil

3 c. spinach

1 c. egg substitute

3 eggs

¼ c. crumbled feta cheese

½ c. shredded mozzarella cheese

2 tbsp. chopped fresh basil

¼ c. rehydrated sun-dried tomatoes

¼ tsp. kosher salt

Ground black pepper to taste

1. Heat the oven to 375 F.
2. Heat a medium sauté pan to medium heat; add olive oil. Sauté spinach until wilted; remove from heat.
3. In a mixing bowl, whisk the eggs and egg substitute. Gradually add the remaining ingredients; mix well.
4. Pour mixture back into a baking pan or the warm sauté pan, stirring it while in the pan. Cover with parchment paper and foil.
5. Bake approximately 20 minutes. When the egg mixture is fairly set, uncover and place frittata back in oven about 5 minutes.
6. Cut into six triangles or squares and serve.

PYRAMID SERVINGS:

PD Protein/Dairy   1

PER SERVING
(1 TRIANGLE OR SQUARE):

Calories	97
Protein	10 g
Carbohydrate	3 g
Total fat	5 g
Cholesterol	103 mg
Sodium	298 mg
Fiber	0.5 g

CHEF'S NOTES:

To make sure the seasoning of the frittata is appropriate, scramble a small amount of it in a heated pan and taste.

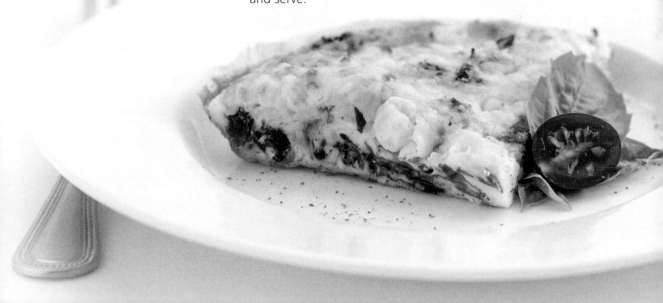

BBQ Chicken Chopped Salad

✦ SERVES 4

- 8 oz. boneless, skinless chicken breast
- 2 tbsp. BBQ sauce
- 8 c. washed and chopped romaine lettuce
- 4 tbsp. chopped fresh cilantro
- 4 tbsp. chopped fresh basil
- ½ c. black beans
- ½ c. frozen sweet corn, thawed
- 2 corn tortillas, 4.5" each, cut into strips, baked in oven until crispy
- 4 tbsp. shredded colby or Monterey Jack cheese
- 3 Roma tomatoes, diced
- ¼ c. chopped green onions
- ½ avocado, sliced
- 4 tbsp. reduced-fat ranch dressing

1. Grill, sear or bake chicken breast until done.
2. Heat the BBQ sauce.
3. Dice the chicken and mix with the BBQ sauce.
4. Mix the lettuce, cilantro and basil together and place in four medium bowls.
5. Divide the black beans and corn evenly among the bowls.
6. Place even amounts of the chicken mixture, cheese, tomatoes and avocado in each bowl. Top with tortilla strips and green onions.
7. Serve 1 tablespoon of ranch dressing with each salad.

PYRAMID SERVINGS:

V	Vegetables	1
C	Carbohydrates	1
PD	Protein/Dairy	1
Ft	Fats	1

PER SERVING
(¼ OF RECIPE - 1 BOWL):

Calories	272
Protein	25 g
Carbohydrate	25 g
Total fat	9 g
Cholesterol	50 mg
Sodium	284 mg
Fiber	7 g

CHEF'S NOTES:

 Keep an easy-open container of corn in the freezer instead of opening a new bag each time. Don't use dried basil or cilantro as a replacement for the fresh varieties. The tortillas are included to add crunch and can be omitted, if desired.

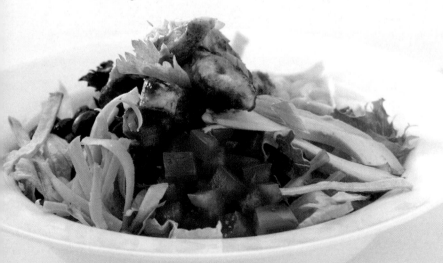

Roasted Red Pepper Pineapple Salsa

✚ SERVES 4

½ c. chopped roasted red bell pepper

1 c. diced pineapple

¼ c. finely chopped fresh cilantro

¼ c. finely chopped red onion

2 tbsp. diced jalapeno pepper

2 tsp. honey

¼ tsp. salt

1. To roast the red pepper, heat a charcoal or gas grill, or set the oven to 425 F.
   Grill: Place the pepper directly on the hot grill, turning every 2 minutes until the skin is blackened.
   Oven: Place the pepper on a grill pan and roast for 15-20 minutes until the skin is blackened.
2. Place the pepper in a bowl and cover it with plastic wrap to create steam; wait 5-10 minutes. Remove the pepper from the bowl, remove the skin and chop the pepper.
3. In a medium bowl, combine all ingredients and mix well. Cover and refrigerate until served.

PYRAMID SERVINGS:

V	Vegetables	0.5
F	Fruits	0.5

PER SERVING (¼ CUP):

Calories	40
Protein	1 g
Carbohydrate	10 g
Total fat	0 g
Cholesterol	0 mg
Sodium	125 mg
Fiber	1 g

CHEF'S NOTES:

You can use other fruits such as oranges, mango or papaya. If you dislike cilantro, use fresh parsley. Roasted red bell peppers sold in stores may be substituted for fresh. The salsa is great on fish, grilled chicken, tofu, pork tenderloin and fajitas.

Shrimp Tostada

✚ SERVES 4

4 corn tortillas (6-inch)

1 c. black beans

1 tsp. cumin

1 tsp. hot pepper sauce

2 tsp. olive oil

8 oz. large shrimp, peeled and deveined, chopped

1 lime, juiced

2 tbsp. chopped cilantro

2 tsp. minced garlic

½ tsp. kosher or sea salt

1 c. shredded romaine lettuce

1 c. diced fresh pineapple

2 Roma tomatoes, chopped

¼ c. crumbled feta cheese

4 green onions, chopped

1. Heat the oven to 375 F.
2. Toast tortillas until crisp, about 15 minutes.
3. In a small sauté pan, heat the beans on medium heat. Add cumin and hot pepper sauce. Smash beans to make a slight puree.
4. Bring another medium-sized sauté pan to medium heat and add oil. When the pan is hot, add shrimp. Add lime juice, cilantro, garlic and salt. Sauté until shrimp are bright red.
5. Place ¼ cup smashed black beans on each tortilla. Top with lettuce, shrimp, pineapple, tomatoes, cheese and green onions.

PYRAMID SERVINGS:

V	Vegetables	0.5
F	Fruits	0.5
C	Carbohydrates	1
PD	Protein/Dairy	1
Ft	Fats	0.5

PER SERVING (1 TOSTADA):

Calories	233
Protein	15 g
Carbohydrate	34 g
Total fat	6 g
Cholesterol	78 mg
Sodium	567 mg
Fiber	6 g

CHEF'S NOTES:

You can substitute soft-shelled tacos for the corn tortillas. You can also substitute grilled or baked chicken for the shrimp.

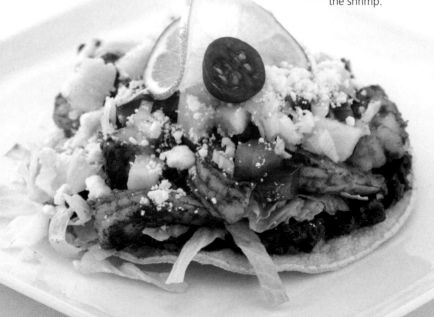

Chicken Salad Sandwich

✛ SERVES 6

3 4-oz. boneless, skinless chicken breasts

¼ tsp. sea salt

¼ tsp. white pepper

¼ tsp. onion powder

1 c. red grapes, cut in half

¼ c. low-fat mayonnaise

¼ c. finely diced celery

¼ c. diced tomato

4 slices turkey bacon, cooked and crumbled

1 tbsp. chopped green onion

2 oz. Swiss or Gruyere cheese, cubed

6 slices whole-wheat bread

Lettuce leaves

Red onion, sliced

1. Heat the oven to 375 F.
2. Season the chicken with salt, pepper and onion powder. Grill or bake until thoroughly cooked to an internal temperature of 165 F.
3. Let chicken cool slightly and chop into medium-sized pieces.
4. In a medium bowl, combine the chicken, grapes, mayonnaise, celery, tomato, bacon, onion and cheese. Refrigerate until ready to serve.
5. To build the sandwiches, place about ½ cup of chicken salad mixture on 3 slices of bread. Top with lettuce and onion and remaining slices of bread. Cut in half before serving.

PYRAMID SERVINGS:

C	Carbohydrates	1
PD	Protein/Dairy	1
Ft	Fats	2

PER SERVING (½ SANDWICH):

Calories	320
Protein	26 g
Carbohydrate	29 g
Total fat	12 g
Cholesterol	84 mg
Sodium	612 mg
Fiber	3.5 g

CHEF'S NOTES:

For this recipe, use only the white bulb portion of the green onion.

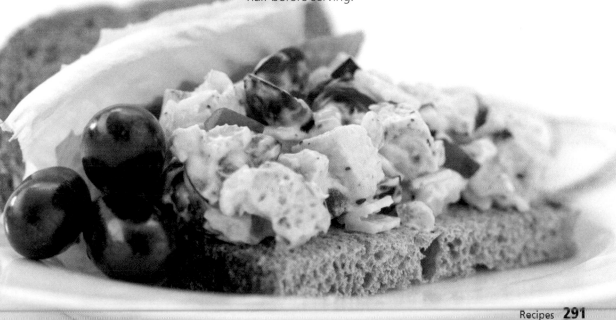

Roasted Butternut Squash Fries

✚ SERVES 6

2 medium butternut squash

1 tbsp. chopped fresh thyme

1 tbsp. chopped fresh
    rosemary

1 tbsp. olive oil

½ tsp. salt

1. Heat the oven to 425 F. Lightly coat a baking sheet with cooking spray. Peel skin from squash and cut into even sticks, about ½-inch wide and 3 inches long.

2. In a medium bowl, combine the squash, thyme, rosemary, oil and salt; mix until the squash is evenly coated. Spread onto the baking sheet and roast for 10 minutes in the oven.

3. Remove the baking sheet from the oven and shake to loosen the squash. Place back in the oven and roast another 5 to 10 minutes until golden brown.

PYRAMID SERVINGS:

V	Vegetables	1
Ft	Fats	0.5

PER SERVING (½ CUP):

Calories	62
Protein	1 g
Carbohydrate	11 g
Total fat	2 g
Cholesterol	0 mg
Sodium	168 mg
Fiber	3 g

CHEF'S NOTES:

This recipe also works well with sweet potatoes or acorn squash. To ensure even cooking, cut the vegetables so all the pieces are similar in size.

Dijon Parmesan Crusted Salmon

✦ SERVES 4

¼ c. Dijon mustard

2 tbsp. low-fat mayonnaise

¼ c. grated Parmesan cheese

¼ c. panko breadcrumbs

4 salmon fillets, each approx. 4 oz.

¼ tsp. salt

¼ tsp. ground black pepper

2 tsp. olive oil

1. Heat the oven to 375 F.
2. In small bowl, combine mustard and mayonnaise. In another bowl, combine cheese and panko.
3. Coat the top of each salmon fillet with 1½ tablespoons mustard mixture, and then cover with 2 tablespoons panko mixture, evened out. Sprinkle each fillet with salt and pepper.
4. Heat a large nonstick pan to medium-high heat; add oil. Place the salmon fillets crusted side down for about 1 minute or until golden brown. Place oven-proof pan in the oven to finish cooking, or place the fillets on a baking sheet crusted side up. Bake about 6 minutes or until the fillets flake with a fork.

PYRAMID SERVINGS:

PD	Protein/Dairy	2
Ft	Fats	1

PER SERVING (4 OUNCES):

Calories	243
Protein	27 g
Carbohydrate	4 g
Total fat	11.5 g
Cholesterol	64 mg
Sodium	718 mg
Fiber	0 g

CHEF'S NOTES:

Tilapia, cod or trout can be substituted for the salmon. Keep a close watch on the cooking time. Fish can become dry if overcooked. When using oil in a frying pan you may need to lower the heat. The cooking time may be longer if heat needs to be lowered.

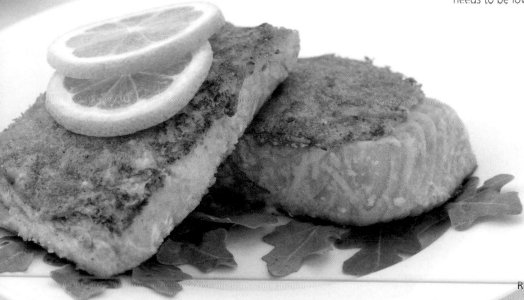

Roasted Vegetables

+ SERVES 6

3 medium zucchini, cut into ½-inch chunks

1½ red onion, cut into ½-inch chunks

1½ red bell pepper, cut into ½-inch chunks

1½ yellow bell pepper or summer squash, cut into ½-inch chunks

6 portobello mushrooms, sliced

⅓ c. chopped fresh parsley

⅓ c. lemon juice

3 garlic cloves, minced

1½ tsp. olive oil

1½ tsp. chopped fresh oregano

¾ tsp. ground black pepper

¼ tsp. sea salt

1. Heat the oven to 400 F. Combine all of the ingredients in a large bowl. Set aside for 10 minutes to marinate.

2. Lightly coat a 15-by-10-inch pan with cooking spray. Arrange vegetables on the pan in a single layer. Roast in the oven for 20 minutes or until vegetables are crisp-tender.

PYRAMID SERVINGS:

V Vegetables	1.5

PER SERVING (¾ CUP):

Calories	70
Protein	3 g
Carbohydrate	13 g
Total fat	2 g
Cholesterol	6 mg
Sodium	81 mg
Fiber	3 g

CHEF'S NOTES:

 Any vegetable can be roasted. If roasting harder vegetables, such as carrots, butternut squash and cauliflower, first steam the vegetables for about a minute.

Quinoa Cakes

✚ SERVES 14

2 large sweet potatoes

2 c. cooked quinoa

2 eggs

3 cloves garlic, minced

6 oz. Gruyere or Parmesan cheese, shredded

2 tbsp. finely chopped fresh parsley

1 tsp. salt

¼ tsp. ground black pepper

¼ tsp. ground nutmeg

2 tbsp. olive oil for searing

1. Heat the oven to 375 F. Spear sweet potatoes with a knife and bake about 45 minutes until soft.
2. Cook the quinoa.
3. Let the sweet potatoes and quinoa cool. Remove the skins from the potatoes and mash.
4. In a large bowl, combine 2 cups mashed potatoes with quinoa, eggs, garlic, cheese, parsley, salt, pepper and nutmeg. Take amounts of approximately ¼-cup and form into patties.
5. Preheat a large sauté pan to medium heat. Added 1 tablespoon olive oil. Cook until cakes are golden brown on each side. Repeat the process with remaining mixture and oil. Bake the cakes in the oven for an additional 5 minutes.

PYRAMID SERVINGS:

C	Carbohydrates	1
PD	Protein/Dairy	0.5
Ft	Fats	1

PER SERVING (1 CAKE):

Calories	123
Protein	6 g
Carbohydrate	10 g
Total fat	6.5 g
Cholesterol	38 mg
Sodium	172 mg
Fiber	1.5 g

CHEF'S NOTES:

If serving as a main meal, two quinoa cakes equate to a meal portion. The cakes can be prepared in advance and frozen for later use.

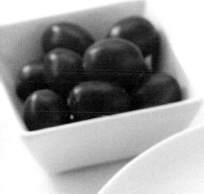

Chicken Sausage Meatballs

✛ SERVES 6

⅓ large onion, finely diced

2½ tsp. garlic, minced

⅓ c. grated Parmesan cheese

1 tsp. Italian seasoning

1 tsp. ground fennel

¼ tsp. kosher salt

⅛ tsp. ground black pepper

1½ lbs. ground chicken breast

1. Heat the oven to 350 F.
2. Lightly coat a baking sheet with cooking spray.
3. In a small saucepan, sauté onions and garlic. Cook until tender, about 5-7 minutes.
4. Remove onions and garlic from heat and place in medium bowl. Add cheese, Italian seasoning, fennel, salt and pepper and mix. Add the ground chicken and combine it with the mixture.
5. Form into 1-inch meatballs (about ¾-ounce each). Place meatballs on the baking sheet and bake for approximately 15 minutes until they reach an internal temperature of 165 F.

PYRAMID SERVINGS:

PD Protein/Dairy	1.5

**PER SERVING
(3 OZ., 3 TO 4 MEATBALLS):**

Calories	220
Protein	37 g
Carbohydrate	3 g
Total fat	5.5 g
Cholesterol	101 mg
Sodium	422 mg
Fiber	0.5 g

CHEF'S NOTES:

These meatballs can be made ahead of time. Chill in the refrigerator overnight to use the next day or freeze in a freezer bag for up to three months. Serve with a small amount of marinara sauce, if desired.

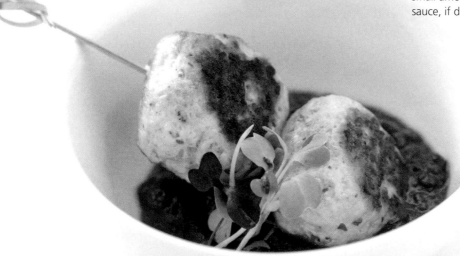

Garlic Mashed Cauliflower Potatoes

✚ SERVES 6

1 to 2 medium russet
potatoes, peeled and
chopped into medium
chunks

3 c. cauliflower florets

1 tbsp. unsalted butter

¼ c. fat-free Greek yogurt

½ tsp. kosher salt

½ tsp. finely chopped fresh
thyme

½ tsp. garlic powder

Ground black pepper to
taste

1. Boil potatoes and cauliflower
   in separate pots until tender.
   Remove from heat and drain.
2. Place the cauliflower in a food
   processor and process until
   smooth, about 2 minutes. Whip
   the potatoes with a mixer on
   medium speed about 1 minute.
3. Add cauliflower to potato
   mixture. Mix slowly while adding
   butter, yogurt, salt, thyme, garlic
   powder and pepper. Mix on
   medium speed about 2 minutes
   until thoroughly combined.

PYRAMID SERVINGS:

V	Vegetables	0.5
C	Carbohydrates	0.5
Ft	Fats	0.5

PER SERVING (½ CUP):

Calories	81
Protein	3 g
Carbohydrate	13 g
Total fat	2 g
Cholesterol	6 mg
Sodium	514 mg
Fiber	2 g

CHEF'S NOTES:

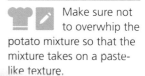 Make sure not
to overwhip the
potato mixture so that the
mixture takes on a paste-
like texture.

Macadamia Nut Crusted Walleye

✚ SERVES 2

6 tbsp. macadamia nuts

6 tbsp. panko breadcrumbs

1 tbsp. chopped fresh parsley

¼ tsp. kosher salt

¼ tsp. garlic powder

¼ tsp. onion powder

Pinch ground black pepper

1 tsp. olive oil

2 walleye fillets, each approx. 4 oz.

CHEF'S NOTES:

This seasoning mixture also can be used on other fish, as well as on poultry and meat.

1. In a food processor, combine nuts and breadcrumbs; pulse to an even consistency.
2. In a small bowl, combine bread-crumb mixture, parsley, salt, garlic powder, onion powder and pepper. Coat the top of each fillet (not the skin side) with half the seasoning mixture.
3. Heat a large sauté pan to medium-high heat; add oil. Sear seasoned side of fillet first, about 1 minute. Carefully flip over and lower heat to medium. Cover and let cook 2-3 minutes, until fillets reach an internal temperature of 145 F. Walleye should flake when it's done.

PYRAMID SERVINGS:

C Carbohydrates		0.5
PD Protein/Dairy		1
Ft Fats		3

PER SERVING (4 OUNCES):

Calories	343
Protein	24 g
Carbohydrate	12 g
Total fat	23.5 g
Cholesterol	95 mg
Sodium	382 mg
Fiber	2.5 g

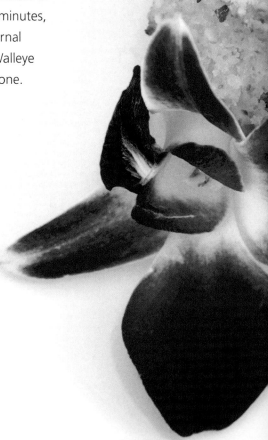

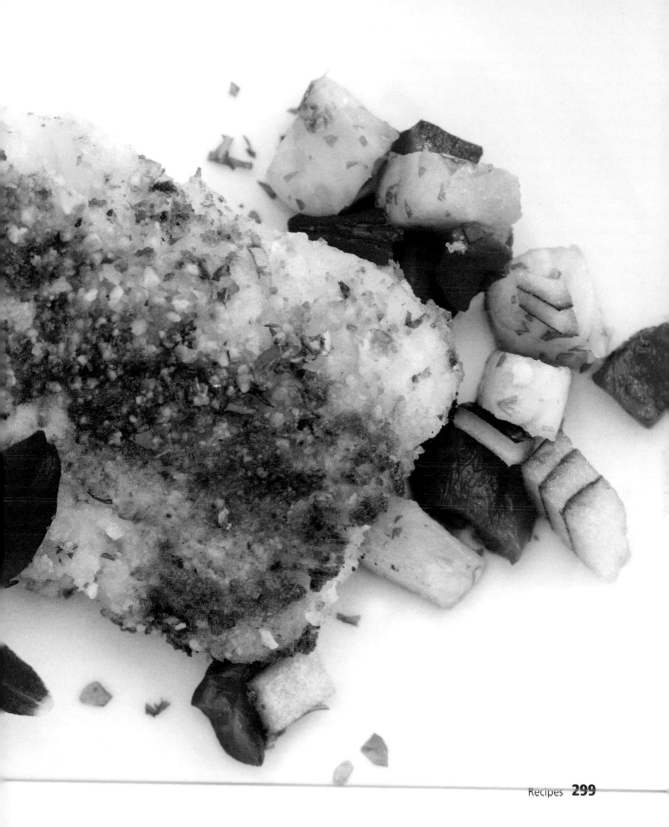

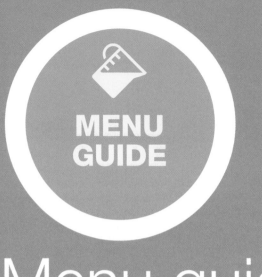

MENU GUIDE

Menu guide

When you eat at home, it's easier to eat healthy foods and control portion sizes. These 1,200-calorie sample menus can help you plan balanced, delicious meals.

The menus provide generous portions of vegetables and fruits, four servings of carbohydrates, three servings of protein and dairy, and three servings of fats. If your daily calorie goal is higher, you'll need to adjust the menus accordingly.

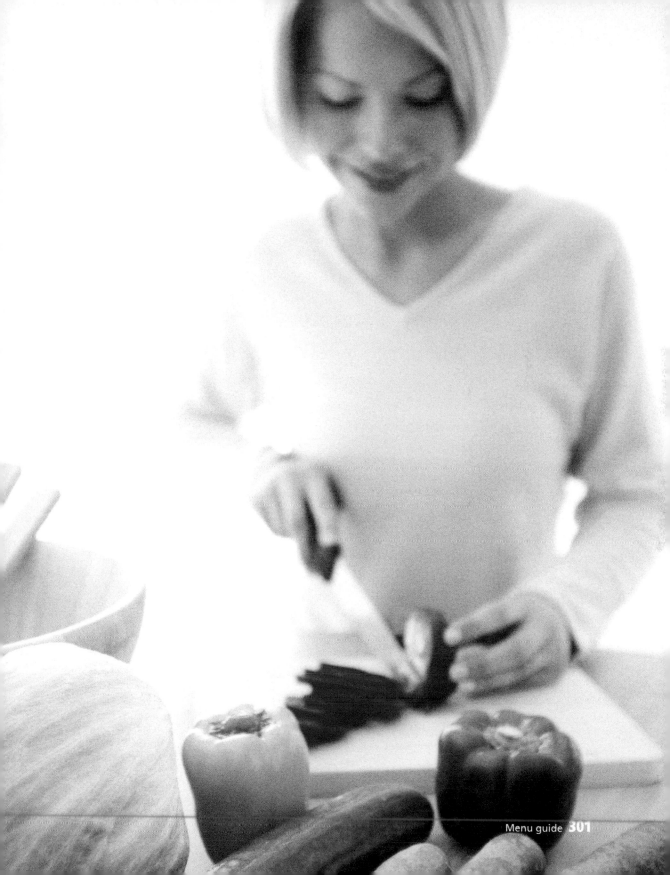

Day 1 menu

Breakfast
+ 1 whole-grain bagel **C** **C**
  (3-inch diameter)
+ 3 tbsp. fat-free cream cheese **Ft**
+ 1 medium orange **F**
+ Calorie-free beverage

Lunch
+ Smoked turkey wrap **C** **PD** **V**
  (Top 6-inch, fat-free tortilla with 3 oz.
  thin-sliced smoked turkey, shredded lettuce, sliced tomato and onion. Top with
  2 tbsp. salsa and roll up.)
+ Cucumber and tomato salad **V**
  (Combine ½ c. thinly sliced cucumber
  and 4 cherry tomatoes, halved. Add balsamic, rice wine or herb-flavored vinegar
  to taste.)
+ 1 small apple **F**
+ Calorie-free beverage

Dinner
+ 3 oz. marinated, broiled flank steak **PD** **PD**
  (Marinate in fat-free Italian dressing.)
+ ½ medium baked potato **C**
+ 2 tbsp. sour cream **Ft**
+ ⅔ c. green beans **V**
+ ¼ small cantaloupe **F**
+ Calorie-free beverage

Snack
+ 1 serving favorite vegetable **V**
+ 3 tbsp. fat-free ranch dressing **Ft**

10 practical steps to healthier eating

1. Have at least one serving of fruit at each meal and one as a snack during the day.
2. Include at least two servings of vegetables at lunch and dinner.
3. Switch from low-fiber breakfast cereal to lower sugar, higher fiber alternatives.
4. Choose whole-grain breads, switch to brown rice instead of white, and when baking, experiment with whole-wheat flour.
5. Lighten your milk by moving down one step in fat content — from whole to 2 percent, for instance, or from 1 percent to skim milk.
6. Cook with olive, canola or another vegetable oil instead of butter or trans fat-free margarine.
7. Flavor foods with herbs and spices rather than sauces and gravies.
8. Have fish at least twice a week.
9. Serve fresh fruit for dessert.
10. Drink calorie-free beverages instead of sugar-sweetened ones.

Week 1

Day 2 menu

Breakfast
+ 1 whole-grain bagel C C
  (3-inch diameter)
+ 3 tbsp. fat-free cream cheese Ft
+ 1 small apple F
+ 1 c. skim milk PD
+ Calorie-free beverage

Lunch
+ 1 c. vegetable soup C
+ 2 c. lettuce, 1 medium tomato
  cut into wedges V V
+ 2 tbsp. fat-free salad dressing Ft
+ 1 c. reduced-calorie, fat-free yogurt
  mixed with ¾ c. berries PD F
+ Calorie-free beverage

Dinner
+ 2½ oz. boneless, skinless chicken
  breast PD
+ 3 red-skinned baby potatoes with
  fresh parsley C
+ 2 c. steamed broccoli V V
+ 2 tsp. trans fat-free margarine-
  like spread Ft
+ Calorie-free beverage

Snack
+ 1 small pear F

> Remember, you can eat unlimited
> servings of vegetables and fruits.

Dietitian's Tips

+ Vary your salad greens to take
advantage of the multitude of
nutrients, flavors and textures.
Butterhead (Boston, or bibb) lettuce
is delicate in texture and flavor.
Loose-leaf lettuce (oak-leaf, red-leaf
or green-leaf) has easily separated
leaves that are flavorful and crisp.
Romaine (cos) lettuce has a crunchy
texture and somewhat bitter taste.

+ Don't be fooled into thinking
"low-calorie" dressings are really low
in calories. Most aren't. According
to labeling laws, a low-calorie salad
dressing may have up to 40 calories
a serving. When possible, choose fat-
free salad dressings. They generally
have 25 calories or less a serving.

+ Salsa isn't only for chips. Try it on
potatoes, vegetables, and as a topping
for fish, chicken or meats.

Day 3 menu

Breakfast
+ 1 c. reduced-calorie, fat-free yogurt **PD**
+ 1 small banana **F**
+ 1 graham cracker **C**
+ Calorie-free beverage

Lunch
+ **Mixed green salad** **V** **V** **V**
  (Combine 2 c. spring mixed greens with ½ tomato, sliced; ½ cucumber, sliced; and red onion.)
+ **2 tbsp. fat-free French dressing** **Ft**
+ **1 small apple** **F**
+ **2 crispy breadsticks** **C**
+ **Calorie-free beverage**

Dinner
+ **Grilled salmon with sliced cucumber and radish** **V** **PD** **Ft**
  See recipe on this page. ✔
+ **1 whole-grain roll** **C**
+ **1 tsp. trans fat-free margarine-like spread** **Ft**
+ **¾ c. berries** **F**
+ **Calorie-free beverage**

Snack
+ **8 wheat crackers** **C**
+ **2 oz. low-fat cheddar cheese** **PD**

Grilled Salmon With Sliced Cucumber and Radish

RECIPE

+ Serves 4

1 lb. salmon fillet

½ tsp. lemon juice

½ tbsp. olive oil

1 c. seeded and thinly sliced cucumber

½ c. thinly sliced radishes

1 tbsp. vinegar

⅛ tsp. dill weed

Ground black pepper, optional

1. Rub salmon with lemon juice and oil. Cut into four pieces. Place salmon, skin-side down onto aluminum foil sprayed with cooking spray.
2. In a bowl combine remaining ingredients and refrigerate.
3. Grill or broil the salmon at medium to high heat until the salmon is flaky but still moist, or an internal temperature of 145 F.
4. Top each piece of salmon with the cucumber and radish mixture.

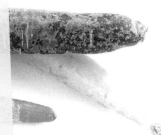

Week 1

Day 4 menu

Breakfast

+ **1 c. whole-grain breakfast cereal** `C` `C`
+ **1 c. skim milk** `PD`
+ **1 medium orange** `F`
+ **Calorie-free beverage**

Lunch

+ **Grilled chicken salad** `V` `V` `PD` `Ft`
  (Combine 2 c. mixed greens with 2½ oz. grilled boneless, skinless chicken breast and 1 c. cherry tomatoes, bell peppers and chopped green onions. Top with 1 tsp. extra-virgin olive oil mixed with 2 tbsp. red wine vinegar. Sprinkle with cracked black pepper.)
+ **1 small pear** `F`
+ **Calorie-free beverage**

Dinner

+ **3 oz. grilled tuna or other fish** `PD`
  (Sprinkle with lemon juice and basil.)
+ **⅔ c. cooked brown rice** `C` `C`
+ **1½ c. steamed summer squash and zucchini** `V` `V`
+ **1 tsp. trans fat-free margarine-like spread** `Ft`
+ **1 c. grapes** `F`
+ **Calorie-free beverage**

Snack

+ **8 whole peanuts** `Ft`

> Remember you can eat unlimited servings of vegetables and fruits.

Self-esteem boosters

How do you feel about yourself? Your answer to that question expresses your level of self-esteem. Here are ways to help you boost your self-esteem and keep a positive attitude:

+ **Change your perspective.** Think about things you do well instead of focusing on what you're unable to do.

+ **Take care of yourself.** Pay attention to both your physical and emotional needs. Set aside time for regular meals, rest and personal hygiene. If you value yourself, others will value you as well.

+ **Exercise.** Setting and accomplishing a physical activity goal can give you an emotional boost, as well as help you achieve a healthy weight.

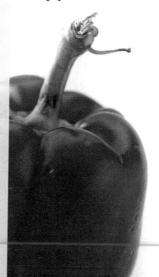

Week 1

Day 5 menu

Week 1

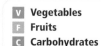

V	Vegetables	**PD**	Protein/Dairy
F	Fruits	**Ft**	Fats
C	Carbohydrates	**S**	Sweets

Breakfast
+ 1 c. whole-grain breakfast cereal **C** **C**
+ 1 c. skim milk **PD**
+ ½ large grapefruit **F**
+ Calorie-free beverage

Lunch
+ Spinach fruit salad **V** **V** **F**
  (Top 2 c. baby spinach leaves with 1 c. green pepper strips and water chestnuts, and ¾ c. mandarin orange sections.)
+ 2 tbsp. fat-free French dressing **Ft**
+ 8 whole-grain crackers **C**
+ 1 c. skim milk **PD**
+ Calorie-free beverage

Dinner
+ 3 oz. lean pork **PD**
+ ½ c. wild rice **C**
+ 1 c. asparagus **V** **V**
+ 2 tsp. trans fat-free margarine-like spread **Ft**
+ Calorie-free beverage

Snack
+ ¾ c. berries **F**
+ ½ c. nondairy whipped topping **Ft**

Remember you can eat unlimited servings of vegetables and fruits.

Dietitian's Tips

+ Choose locally grown fruit that's in season. Generally, the closer you are to the growing source, the fresher the produce and the better it tastes.

+ Select fruits that feel heavy for their size. Heaviness is a sign of juiciness.

+ Keep fruits at room temperature to ripen them. Fruits such as bananas, pears, nectarines and kiwi are often picked and sold at grocery stores before they're ripe.

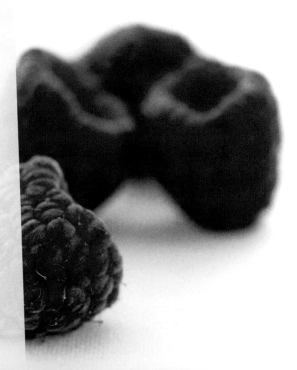

Day 6 menu

Breakfast

+ 1 egg, fried in nonstick pan **PD**
+ 1 slice whole-grain toast **C**
+ 2 tsp. trans fat-free margarine-like spread **Ft**
+ ½ c. orange juice **F**
+ Calorie-free beverage

Lunch

+ Roast beef sandwich **V** **PD** **C** **C**
  (Fill 1 whole-grain roll with 1½ oz. sliced lean roast beef, Dijon mustard, lettuce, tomato and red onion slices.)
+ ½ c. baby carrots **V**
+ 1 c. grapes **F**
+ Calorie-free beverage

Dinner

+ Shrimp stir-fry **PD** **V** **Ft**
  See recipe on this page. ✔
+ ⅓ c. cooked brown rice **C**
+ 2 c. mixed greens **V**
+ 2 tbsp. reduced-calorie salad dressing **Ft**
+ Calorie-free beverage

Snack

+ 1 serving favorite fruit **F**

Shrimp Stir-Fry
+ Serves 4

1-2 cloves garlic, chopped

⅛ tsp. grated or finely chopped fresh ginger

1 tbsp. olive oil

2½ c. (about ½ lb.) fresh sugar snap peas

½ c. chopped red bell sweet pepper (optional)

12 oz. medium-sized raw shrimp,
   peeled and deveined

1. Sauté garlic and ginger in oil in large skillet until fragrant.
2. Stir in snap peas and chopped bell pepper, if desired. Sauté until tender-crisp.
3. Stir in shrimp. Cook over medium heat 3 to 4 minutes until shrimp are opaque in the center.
4. Serve immediately with rice.

Week 1

Day 7 menu

Breakfast

+ **Breakfast burrito** C C V PD

   (Place ½ c. chopped tomato, 2 tbsp. chopped onion and ¼ c. canned corn in small skillet. Cook until soft. Add egg substitute and scramble with the vegetables until cooked through. Place mixture in center of whole-wheat tortilla, top with salsa, fold and eat.)

+ **1 medium orange** F
+ **Calorie-free beverage**

Lunch

+ **Turkey pita sandwich** V C PD Ft

   (Stuff ½ whole-grain pita with 3 oz. shredded turkey, ⅙ avocado, chopped lettuce, tomato and onion.)

+ **1 small apple** F
+ **Calorie-free beverage**

Dinner

+ **Tuna-stuffed tomato** PD V Ft Ft

   (Drain and mix 3 oz. water-packed tuna with 4 tsp. regular mayonnaise. Season with black pepper and a bit of chopped pickle, if desired. Core and partially quarter a tomato. Stuff it with tuna mixture.)

+ **4 medium celery sticks** V
+ **6 wheat crackers** C
+ **Calorie-free beverage**

Snack

+ **1 serving favorite fruit** F

5 ways to add physical activity to your day

1. Take the stairs instead of the elevator or escalator for at least a few floors.

2. Walk or bike to nearby destinations instead of always driving.

3. Get off the bus a few blocks early or park three blocks from work.

4. Exercise while watching television.

5. Do housework, such as vacuuming, washing the floors, polishing the furniture or washing the windows.

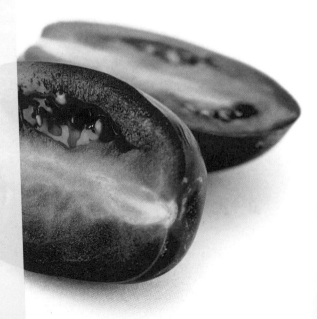

Week 1

Day 8 menu

Breakfast
+ **1 c. reduced-calorie, fat-free yogurt** PD
+ **1 c. pineapple chunks** F F
  (unsweetened, drained)
+ **Calorie-free beverage**

Lunch
+ **Ham sandwich** PD C C
  (Top 2 slices whole-grain bread with 3 oz. lean ham, Dijon mustard, lettuce and tomato slices.)
+ **2 c. mixed salad greens** V
+ **2 tbsp. fat-free French dressing** Ft
+ **Calorie-free beverage**

Dinner
+ **Pasta primavera** PD V V Ft C C
  (Toss 1 c. cooked whole-grain pasta topped with 1 c. steamed carrots, broccoli and cauliflower. Sprinkle with 1 tsp. olive oil and ¼ c. shredded Parmesan cheese.)
+ **1 medium orange** F
+ **Calorie-free beverage**

Snack
+ **1 serving favorite vegetable** V
+ **4 tbsp. fat-free sour cream dip** Ft

Dietitian's Tips

+ Calories from beverages can add up. To cut calories, switch to low-fat or skim milk, drink lower calorie juices, and switch to diet soda.

+ You can dilute juices with plain or sparkling water to reduce calories, too. Add a twist of lemon or lime to perk up your water.

Week 2

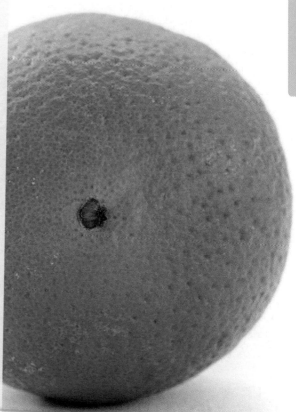

Day 9 menu

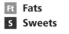

V Vegetables	**PD** Protein/Dairy
F Fruits	**Ft** Fats
C Carbohydrates	**S** Sweets

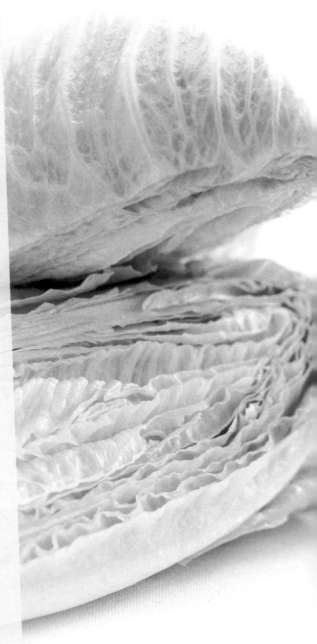

Breakfast

+ **Fruit yogurt parfait** F PD
  (Combine 1 c. reduced-calorie, fat-free vanilla yogurt with 1 c. favorite fruit.)
+ **½ whole-grain bagel** C
  (3-inch diameter)
+ **3 tbsp. fat-free cream cheese** Ft
+ **Calorie-free beverage**

Lunch

+ **Chicken wrap** F C PD S
  (Combine 2½ oz. shredded cooked chicken, 1 tbsp. raisins, 3 tbsp. cranberry sauce and shredded lettuce. Wrap in a 6-inch corn tortilla.)
+ **1 tomato and 1 c. cucumber slices** V V Ft
  (Drizzle with 1 tsp. olive oil and sprinkle with dill to taste.)
+ **Calorie-free beverage**

Dinner

+ **3 oz. marinated pork tenderloin** PD
  (Marinate pork tenderloin in ¼ c. teriyaki sauce for 4 hours, turning frequently. Grill pork, turning occasionally, until thermometer in center of pork reads at least 145 F.)
+ **1 c. asparagus** V V
+ **3 red-skinned baby potatoes** C
+ **1 small whole-grain roll** C
+ **1 tsp. margarine** Ft

Snack

+ **1 serving favorite fruit** F

Week 2

Day 10 menu

Breakfast
+ ½ c. whole-grain cereal **C**
+ 1 c. skim milk **PD**
+ 1 medium orange **F**
+ Calorie-free beverage

Lunch
+ 2 oz. low-fat cheddar cheese **PD**
+ 8 whole-grain snack crackers **C**
+ 1 c. raw baby carrots **V V**
+ 3 tbsp. fat-free ranch dressing **Ft**
+ 1 c. grapes **F**
+ Calorie-free beverage

Dinner
+ 3 oz. grilled halibut or other fish **PD**
+ 1 serving brown rice with vegetables
  C V Ft *See recipe on this page.* ✔
+ 1 c. steamed broccoli with lemon **V**
+ ¾ c. blueberries **F**
+ Calorie-free beverage

Snack
+ 30 pretzel sticks **C**
+ 4 tbsp. fat-free sour
  cream dip **Ft**

Remember you can eat unlimited servings of vegetables and fruits.

Brown Rice With Vegetables
+ Serves 4

1 c. brown rice, uncooked

1 tbsp. olive oil

2 c. reduced-sodium chicken broth (or water)

4 scallions (green onions including tops)

2 c. total — chopped red, green or yellow bell peppers, celery, mushrooms, asparagus, peapods or carrots

2 tbsp. lemon juice

Optional: ground black pepper and chopped fresh parsley

1. In a large saucepan, over medium heat, sauté the rice in the oil for about 2 minutes, stirring frequently. Reduce heat, slowy add broth, cover and simmer about 30 minutes.
2. Chop scallions into small pieces. Do the same with your choice of vegetables.
3. When rice has cooked 30 minutes, add the vegetables and lemon juice. Stir well to combine. Cover and continue to cook until rice is tender but still has some texture (about 10 to 15 minutes more).
4. Season with black pepper and chopped fresh parsley, if desired, and serve.

Day 11 menu

V Vegetables		**PD** Protein/Dairy	
F Fruits		**Ft** Fats	
C Carbohydrates		**S** Sweets	

Breakfast
+ ½ whole-grain bagel **C**
  (3-inch diameter)
+ 1½ tbsp. jam **S**
+ 1 large grapefruit **F** **F**
+ Calorie-free beverage

Lunch
+ Salad **V** **V** **PD** **Ft**
  (Top 2 c. romaine lettuce with ¼ c. diced cucumber, ¼ c. diced red bell pepper, ¼ c. diced carrots, ¼ c. low-fat feta cheese, 1 slice red onion, 2 sliced black olives and 2 pepperoncini peppers. Drizzle with 1 tsp. olive oil and balsamic vinegar to taste.)
+ 8 wheat crackers **C**

Dinner
+ Turkey burger **C** **C** **V** **PD** **PD** **Ft**
  (Top 3 oz. grilled lean ground turkey patty with ½ grilled onion, lettuce and tomato slices. Serve on a small whole-grain bun spread with 2 tsp. mayonnaise.)
+ 1 medium orange **F**
+ Calorie-free beverage

Snack
+ 1 serving favorite vegetable **V**
+ 3 tbsp. fat-free ranch dressing **Ft**

> Remember you can eat unlimited servings of vegetables and fruits.

Menu-planning tips

+ **Keep menus practical and simple.** But, at the same time, don't exclude good flavor and fun. Remember that you need to enjoy your meals if you're expecting to stick with your plan.

+ **Aim for balance.** Try to include at least one serving from most food groups in most meals. To get plenty of vegetables each day, build lunches and dinners that incorporate two vegetable servings each, or have them for snacks during the day.

+ **Don't make meat the focus.** Build the main part of your meal around vegetables and fruits, in addition to rice, or other whole grains and pasta.

+ **Be flexible.** Don't get hung up on hitting exact daily serving totals. Think in terms of the week as well as day to day. If on Monday you don't reach your target for fruit servings, you can add an extra serving or two on Tuesday.

Week 2

Day 12 menu

Breakfast

+ **Blueberry pancake** F C Ft S
  (Top a 4-inch-diameter pancake with ¾ c. blueberries, 1 tsp. trans fat-free margarine-like spread and 1½ tbsp. syrup.)
+ **1 c. skim milk** PD
+ **Calorie-free beverage**

Lunch

+ **Banana and peanut butter bagel** F C C Ft Ft
  (Spread 1 tbsp. peanut butter on a 3-inch-diameter whole-grain bagel and top with 1 small banana, sliced.)
+ **4 stalks celery** V
+ **1 c. fat-free, reduced-calorie yogurt** PD
+ **1 c. grapes** F
+ **Calorie-free beverage**

Dinner

+ **¼ recipe beef stir-fry** PD V
  (Sauté chopped garlic and ginger in 1 tsp. oil. Add ½ pound thin strips of flank steak, scallions, 2 c. green beans sliced diagonally, and ¼ c. soy sauce mixed with 2 tbsp. cornstarch to thicken.)
+ **⅓ c. cooked brown rice** C
+ **6 steamed asparagus spears** V
+ **Calorie-free beverage**

Snack

+ **1 serving favorite vegetable** V

Dietitian's Tips

+ Frozen berries (strawberries, raspberries, blueberries) can be used in place of fresh berries. However, don't expect the same appearance and texture.

+ Fresh vegetables generally provide the best texture and taste, but if you don't have access to fresh vegetables, it's OK to use frozen vegetables. Canned vegetables also may be substituted, but watch for added salt or sugar.

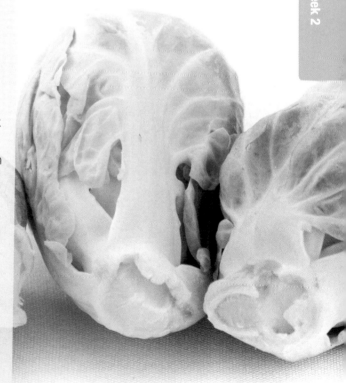

Week 2

Day 13 menu

Breakfast
+ 1 slice whole-grain toast **C**
+ 1 tbsp. peanut butter **Ft** **Ft**
+ 1 medium orange **F**
+ Calorie-free beverage

Lunch
+ ⅔ c. low-fat cottage cheese **PD**
+ 1½ c. strawberries **F**
+ 8 whole-wheat crackers **C**
+ 4 oz. low-sodium vegetable juice **V**
+ Calorie-free beverage

Dinner
+ 1 serving baked chicken and wild rice with onion and tarragon **V** **V** **PD** **C** **C**
  See recipe on this page. ✔
+ 2 tsp. trans fat-free margarine-like spread **Ft**
+ ⅔ c. green beans **V**
+ 1 c. raspberries **F**
+ Calorie-free beverage

Snack
+ 1 c. reduced-calorie, low-fat yogurt **PD**

Baked Chicken and Wild Rice With Onion and Tarragon
+ Serves 6

6 chicken breast halves

1½ c. chopped celery

1½ c. whole pearl onions

1 tsp. fresh tarragon

2 c. unsalted chicken broth

1½ c. dry white wine

1 package long grain and wild rice mix and seasoning packet

1. Heat the oven to 300 F.

2. Remove skin and bones from chicken breasts and cut into ½- to 1-inch pieces. Combine the chicken, celery, pearl onions and tarragon plus 1 c. unsalted chicken broth in a nonstick frying pan. Cook on medium heat until the chicken and vegetables are tender, about 10 minutes. Set aside to cool.

3. In a baking dish, combine the wine, remaining 1 cup chicken broth, rice and seasoning packet. Let soak for 30 minutes.

4. Add the cooked chicken and vegetables to the baking dish. Cover and bake for 60 minutes. Check periodically and add more broth if the rice is too dry.

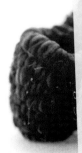

Day 14 menu

Breakfast

+ ½ large grapefruit **F**
+ 1 slice whole-wheat toast **C**
+ 2 tsp. trans fat-free margarine-like spread **Ft**
+ Calorie-free beverage

Lunch

+ **Southwestern salad** **F** **V** **V** **Ft** **Ft** **PD**
  (Top 2 c. shredded lettuce with 2½ oz. shredded cooked chicken, 1 c. chopped green peppers and onions, ⅓ c. crushed pineapple, ⅙ avocado, and 3 tbsp. reduced-calorie Western-style salad dressing.)
+ Calorie-free beverage

Dinner

+ 4 oz. large shrimp, steamed **PD**
+ ⅔ c. cooked brown rice **C** **C**
+ 1½ c. zucchini and summer squash, steamed **V** **V**
+ 1 medium peach **F**
+ Calorie-free beverage

Snack

+ 2 oz. low-fat cheddar cheese **PD**
+ 8 whole-wheat crackers **C**

Remember you can eat unlimited servings of vegetables and fruits.

Dietitian's Tips

Dishes prepared with boneless, skinless chicken are frequent offerings in a healthy diet. Here are simple ways to vary your menu.

Seasonings to use with chicken:
+ Barbecue sauce
+ Chili sauce
+ Curry powder
+ Dijon-style mustard and honey
+ Garlic-herb or lemon-herb blend
+ Italian seasoning
+ Taco seasoning
+ Tarragon and lemon juice
+ Teriyaki or soy sauce

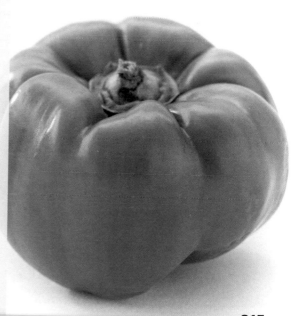

Day 15 menu

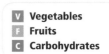

V	Vegetables	PD	Protein/Dairy
F	Fruits	Ft	Fats
C	Carbohydrates	S	Sweets

Breakfast

+ **Blueberry muffin** C Ft
  See recipe on page 285. ✔
+ **1 c. reduced calorie, fat-free yogurt** PD
+ **1 medium peach** F
+ **Calorie-free beverage**

Lunch

+ **Turkey pita** Ft C PD
  (½ pita, 3 oz. white turkey meat,
  1 lettuce leaf, 1 slice red onion,
  ½ tomato, ¼ tsp. balsamic vinegar)
+ **Salad** V Ft F
  (2 c. arugula, ½ c. pomegranates,
  ½ c. vegetables of choice)
+ **Calorie-free beverage**

Dinner

+ **1 c. spaghetti with meatballs and tomato sauce** V V C PD Ft
+ **1 garlic breadstick with cheese** C PD Ft
+ **Calorie-free beverage**

Snack

+ **1 small apple** F
+ **1½ tsp. peanut butter** Ft

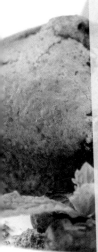

Self-esteem boosters

Here's a scenario: You come home from work starving with no plan of what to cook for dinner. You enter the kitchen to find a cluttered counter top with a dish of candy smack dab in the middle! What might you do in this situation?

If you guessed eat the candy, you're right. Studies show that our food environment — what we keep handy in the kitchen — has an impact on our weight and our overall health. We're three times more likely to consume whatever is in front of us.

To improve your food environment and prevent a hit to your self-esteem:

+ Keep a bowl of fruit or vegetables on the counter so it's the first thing you see.
+ Package snacks such as nuts, veggies or dried fruit in baggies so you can easily grab them when you're hungry.
+ Keep tempting foods, such as candy, out of sight. Better yet, keep them out of the house.

Week 3

Day 16 menu

Breakfast

+ **Egg and spinach sandwich** C PD PD
  (Top 1 whole-wheat English muffin with
  1 egg, ¼ c. spinach, 2 slices tomato)
+ **2 clementines** F
+ **Calorie-free beverage**

Lunch

+ **Southwest wrap** V F C PD Ft
  (Place 2½ oz. shredded chicken, ¼ c. bell
  pepper, ½ c. lettuce, ¼ c. onion, ¼ c.
  salsa and ⅙ avocado on a 6-inch whole-
  wheat flour tortilla)
+ **Roasted butternut squash fries** V F
  See recipe on page 292. ✔
+ **½ c. diced mango** F
+ **Calorie-free beverage**

Dinner

+ **3 oz. broiled cod or other fish** PD
+ **3 baby red potatoes** C
+ **1½ tsp. margarine** Ft F
+ **⅔ c. roasted green beans and
  ½ c. cherry tomatoes** V F
+ **Calorie-free beverage**

Snack

+ **15 cherries** F

**Remember you can eat unlimited
servings of vegetables and fruits.**

5 ways to make sure you stay hydrated

Having enough to drink throughout
the day decreases your risk of dehy-
dration. Staying well-hydrated may
also help you feel more energized
and even reduce your hunger.

How much fluid you need each
day depends on a number of factors,
including your body size and health,
how active you are, and where you
live. A common rule of thumb is
to drink eight 8-ounce glasses of
water a day. This amount is easy to
remember and close to recommendations from health agencies.

To make sure you drink enough
fluids throughout the day:

1. Carry a water bottle with you.
2. Drink water before, during and
after physical activity.
3. Drink water before, during and
after meals.
4. Add fruit to water to make it
more fun and refreshing.
5. Set a timer to remind you to drink
something.

Day 17 menu

V Vegetables	**PD** Protein/Dairy
F Fruits	**Ft** Fats
C Carbohydrates	**S** Sweets

Breakfast
+ 1 slice whole-wheat toast **C**
+ 1½ tsp. peanut butter **Ft**
+ 1 c. blueberries **F**
+ Calorie-free beverage

Lunch
+ **Turkey and cheese sandwich** **C** **C** **PD**
  (2 slices whole-wheat bread,
  2 oz. turkey, 1 oz. low-fat Swiss
  cheese, 1 tsp. Dijon mustard)
+ **Salad** **V** **V**
  (2 c. mixed greens; ½ tomato, sliced;
  ¼ cucumber, sliced; ¼ red onion, sliced)
+ 2 tbsp. fat-free French dressing **Ft**
+ 1 small apple **F**
+ Calorie-free beverage

Dinner
+ **Dijon Parmesan crusted salmon** **PD** **PD** **Ft**
  See recipe on page 293. ✔
+ ½ c. roasted asparagus and
  1 c. mushrooms **V** **V**
+ ½ c. wild rice **C**
+ Calorie-free beverage

Snack
+ 1 small pear **F**

Remember you can eat unlimited
servings of vegetables and fruits.

Dietitian's Tips

Nut butters are made by processing
various nuts into spreads. Peanut
butter is a common example, but
other nuts also make great butters,
such as walnuts, almonds and
pistachios.

You can find nut butters in most
grocery stores, or you can throw
your favorite nuts into a food processor to create your own!

+ **Peanut butter.** It has the
highest amount of protein per
serving at 7g of protein per 2
tablespoons.
+ **Walnut butter.** It has the
greatest amount of healthy
omega-3 fatty acids, which may
help reduce inflammation and
your risk of heart disease.
+ **Almond butter.** Almonds are
highest in fiber and lowest in
saturated fat compared to other
nuts.
+ **Pistachio butter.** Pistachios
contain a significant amount
of an antioxidant called lutein,
which may reduce your risk of
heart disease.

Week 3

Day 18 menu

Breakfast
+ 1 c. reduced-calorie, fat-free yogurt **PD**
+ 1½ c. strawberries **F**
+ ½ whole-grain English muffin **C**
+ 1½ tsp. peanut butter **Ft**
+ Calorie-free beverage

Lunch
+ 3 oz. vegetarian burger patty **PD**
+ 1 whole-grain bun (add lettuce, onion and tomato) **C**
+ 1 tsp. regular mayonnaise **Ft**
+ Roasted vegetables **V Ft**
  See recipe on page 294. ✔
+ 1 c. cantaloupe **F**
+ Calorie-free beverage

Dinner
+ 1 slice (⅛ medium) cheese pizza **V C PD Ft**
+ 2 c. tossed salad with ½ c. chopped vegetables of choice **V Ft**
+ 2 tbsp. fat-free Italian dressing **Ft**
+ 1 c. grapes **F**
+ Calorie-free beverage

Snack
+ 3 c. plain air-popped popcorn **C**

Dietitian's Tips

You may have heard the term *ancient grains*. What are ancient grains? They're whole grains that haven't changed drastically over the past hundred years. This would include whole wheat and wild rice. However, many people think of other grain products when they consider ancient grains, such as quinoa, amaranth, farro, blue corn and einkorn.

Whole grains and whole-grain products, including whole-wheat bread and whole-wheat pasta, are just as healthy as some of the lesser-known ancient grains.

To add variety to your diet, experiment with ancient grains in some of your meals!

Week 3

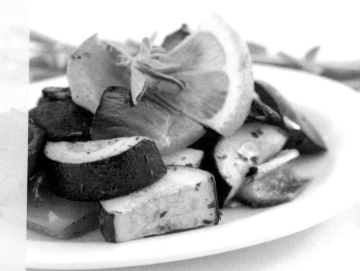

Day 19 menu

V	Vegetables	PD	Protein/Dairy
F	Fruits	Ft	Fats
C	Carbohydrates	S	Sweets

Breakfast

+ **Western omelet** V PD
  (1 egg, ¼ c. chopped onion, ½ green bell pepper, chopped, ¼ c. mushrooms)
+ **½ whole-grain bagel** C
+ **3 tbsp. fat-free cream cheese** Ft
+ **1 small tangerine** F
+ **Calorie-free beverage**

Lunch

+ **Peanut butter and banana sandwich** F C C Ft Ft
  (2 slices of whole-wheat bread, 1 tbsp. peanut butter, 1 small banana)
+ **1 c. sugar snap peas** V F
+ **⅔ c. low-fat cottage cheese** PD
+ **Calorie-free beverage**

Dinner

+ **2½ oz. grilled chicken breast** PD
+ **Roasted red pepper pineapple salsa** Ft Ft
  See recipe on page 289. ✔
+ **⅓ c. brown rice** C
+ **½ c. Brussels sprouts** V
+ **Calorie-free beverage**

Snack

+ **1 large kiwi** F

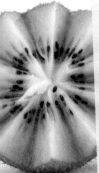

Dietitian's Tips

Cross-utilizing ingredients in the kitchen means having ingredients on hand that can be used in a number of recipes. This saves you time, and it can decrease food waste because each ingredient has several purposes.

An example of cross-utilization is seasoning mixes prepared ahead of time that you can use when needed. Store the mixes in an airtight container to keep them fresh.

Here's one seasoning mix you might want to have handy. You can find recipes for other seasoning mixes on page 187.

Southwest Taco Seasoning
+ Serves 12 (1 serving = 1 tbsp.)

3 tbsp. paprika

3 tbsp. cumin

1½ tbsp. garlic powder

1½ tbsp. onion powder

1½ tbsp. salt

1 tbsp. chili powder

1 tbsp. oregano

1 tbsp. cayenne powder

Week 3

Day 20 menu

Breakfast

+ ¾ c. hot whole-grain cereal C 🔥
+ 1 small banana F
+ Calorie-free beverage

Lunch

+ **Tossed salad** V V 🔥 PD PD
  (2 c. romaine lettuce, ¼ onion, ¼ c. mushrooms, 1 medium tomato, 1 hard-boiled egg, ½ c. low-fat shredded cheddar cheese)
+ **1 whole-wheat dinner roll** C
+ **1½ tsp. butter** Ft 🔥
+ **½ c. cubed pineapple** F
+ **Calorie-free beverage**

Dinner

+ **3 oz. seared scallops in 1 tsp. olive oil** PD Ft
+ **Garlic mashed cauliflower potatoes** 🔥 🔥🔥

  See recipe on page 297. ✔
+ **½ c. beets** V
+ **Calorie-free beverage**

Snack

+ **2 plums** F
+ **8 wheat crackers** C

> Remember you can eat unlimited servings of vegetables and fruits.

Self-esteem boosters

Many of us eat for reasons that aren't related to hunger. We eat because we're distracted, frustrated, stressed or bored. Or we eat because eating has become a trained response — an automatic behavior when we're having a cup of coffee, sitting in traffic or watching a movie.

Before you reach for a snack, ask yourself, "Am I really hungry?" Signs and symptoms of hunger include:

+ Hunger pangs, growling
+ An empty or hollow feeling in your stomach
+ Queasiness

Day 21 menu

V	Vegetables	PD	Protein/Dairy
F	Fruits	Ft	Fats
C	Carbohydrates	S	Sweets

Breakfast
+ 1 c. whole-grain breakfast cereal **C** **C**
+ 1 c. skim milk **PD**
+ 1 c. blackberries **F**
+ Calorie-free beverage

Lunch
+ Chicken salad sandwich **C** **PD** **Ft** **Ft**
  See recipe on page 291. ✔
+ ½ c. baby carrots **V**
+ 4 medium celery stalks **V**
+ 1 c. honeydew melon **F**
+ Calorie-free beverage

Dinner
+ 3 oz. boneless pork chop **PD**
  (Season with ½ tsp. black pepper,
  ½ tsp. cumin, ½ tsp. coriander,
  ½ tsp. cayenne pepper, ¼ tsp.
  garlic powder, ¼ tsp. salt)
+ ¾ c. roasted zucchini **V**
+ 1 tsp. margarine **Ft**
+ 1 small broiled apple (sprinkled
  with cinnamon) **F**
+ Calorie-free beverage

Snack
+ ¼ c. salsa **V**
+ 4 whole-wheat pita chips **C**

Dietitian's **Tips**

To broil an apple:
+ Choose a sweet, firm apple. Peel
and core it and cut it into wedges.
+ Toss the wedges in lemon
juice and arrange them on a
baking sheet.
+ Place the baking sheet about
8 inches from the heat and broil
the wedges for 6 to 8 minutes or
until tender.
+ Remove the wedges from
the oven and sprinkle them
with cinnamon.

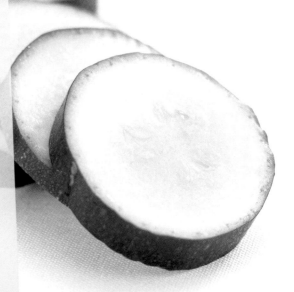

Week 3

Day 22 menu

Breakfast

+ **1 serving sun-dried tomato basil frittata** PD
  See recipe on page 287. ✔
+ **1 slice whole-wheat toast** C
+ **2 tsp. margarine** Ft
+ **¾ c. mixed berries** F
+ **5½ oz. low-sodium vegetable juice** V

Lunch

+ **¼ recipe southwestern chicken and pasta** V V C PD Ft
  See recipe on this page. ✔
+ **1 apple** F
+ **Calorie-free beverage**

Dinner

+ **1 serving shrimp tostada** V F C PD F
  See recipe on page 290. ✔
+ **¼ c. avocado salsa** F
  (1 avocado, cubed; 2 Roma tomatoes, chopped; ⅛ of red onion, chopped; 1 tbsp. chopped cilantro, and 1 clove garlic, minced. Place ingredients in a medium bowl and combine. Squeeze the juice from 1 lime into the bowl, season with pepper and a pinch of salt.)
+ **2 clementines** F
+ **Calorie-free beverage**

Snack

+ **3 c. air-popped popcorn** C

> Remember you can eat unlimited servings of vegetables and fruits.

Southwestern Chicken and Pasta

+ Serves 6

1 c. uncooked pasta

2 (4-oz.) skinless chicken breasts

¼ c. salsa

1½ c. unsalted tomato sauce

⅛ tsp. garlic powder

1 tsp. cumin

½ tsp. chili powder

½ c. canned black beans, rinsed and drained

½ c. fresh or canned corn

¼ c. shredded colby jack (colby and Monterey Jack) cheese

⅙ avocado

1. Cook pasta until tender.
2. Sauté chicken until browned and cooked through, about 10 minutes. Cool slightly and cut chicken into cubes.
3. Stir in the rest of the ingredients along with the cooked pasta. Serve with ⅙ of avocado.

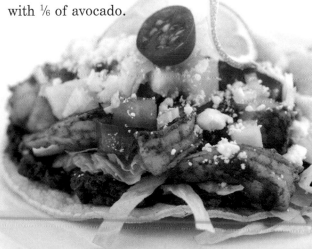

Day 23 menu

Breakfast

+ **Refrigerator oatmeal** F C PD Ft
  (In a bowl or container, combine
  ¼ c. rolled oats, ⅓ c. skim milk,
  ¼ c. low-fat plain Greek yogurt,
  1½ tsp. chia seeds, ¼ c. unsweetened
  applesauce, ¼ c. diced apples, ¼ tsp.
  cinnamon and 1 tsp. honey. Mix well,
  refrigerate overnight, and eat it in the
  morning.)
+ **Calorie-free beverage**

Lunch

+ **Tomato basil pita** V C PD
  (½ whole-wheat pita filled with 1 oz.
  provolone cheese, 1 leaf romaine lettuce, 3 fresh basil leaves, 1 tomato slice,
  1 slice red onion, salt and pepper)
+ **1 c. sugar snap peas** V
+ **1 peach** F
+ **Calorie-free beverage**

Dinner

+ **BBQ chicken chopped salad** V C PD Ft
  See recipe on page 288. ✔
+ **1 whole-grain baguette** C
+ **2 tsp. margarine** Ft
+ **1 banana** F
+ **Calorie-free beverage**

Snack

+ **Vegetable of your choice** V

Dietitian's Tips

Chia seeds are edible seeds that
come from the desert plant *Salvia
hispanica*, which is grown in
Central and South America and
dates back to the Mayan and Aztec
cultures.

The seeds are popular in recipes
because they contain omega-3
fatty acids, carbohydrate, fiber,
protein and antioxidants. One
tablespoon of chia seeds contains
60 calories (40 calories coming
from heart-healthy fats) and 5
grams of fiber. That's 20 percent
of the daily recommended fiber
for women, and 14 percent of the
recommended amount for men.

Chia seeds have a mild, nutty
flavor, and they add a crunchy
texture to cereals, yogurt and
smoothies. The seeds can be
mixed with liquid to form a
gel, similar to tapioca
pudding. Chia seeds can
be found in some recipes for
jams, cereals, baked goods,
puddings and beverages.

Week 4

Day 24 menu

Breakfast
+ **Whole-wheat English muffin with ½ c. cooked egg whites, 1 slice tomato and ¼ c. spinach leaves** `V` `C` `C` `PD`
+ **1 c. cubed honeydew melon** `F`
+ **Calorie-free beverage**

Lunch
+ **½ turkey sandwich** `V` `C` `PD` `Ft`
  (1 slice whole-grain bread, 4 oz. turkey, 1 romaine lettuce leaf, 1 tomato slice, 2 tsp. regular mayonnaise)
+ **1 small apple** `F`
+ **Calorie-free beverage**

Dinner
+ **Southwest taco salad** `V` `V` `C` `PD` `P` `Ft` `Ft`
  See recipe on this page. ✔
+ **¼ c. salsa** `V`
+ **Calorie-free beverage**

Snack
+ **1 small pear** `F`

Remember you can eat unlimited servings of vegetables and fruits.

Southwest Taco Salad

+ Serves 1

¼ c. quinoa

½ c. water

1 c. chopped bell pepper

1 poblano pepper, chopped

3 oz. turkey breast

¼ c. black beans

1 tbsp. low-sodium taco seasoning

1 c. chopped romaine lettuce

2 tsp. lime juice

2 tbsp. shredded sharp cheddar cheese

⅙ avocado

2 tbsp. sour cream

1. Cook quinoa with ½ c. water, according to package instructions.

2. Spray small pan with cooking spray and sauté peppers. Set peppers aside. Brown the turkey breast until cooked through.

3. Add black beans, taco seasoning and lime juice to the pan. Add the quinoa.

4. Place the lettuce in a bowl, then the turkey breast mixture, followed by the sautéed peppers, cheddar cheese, avocado and sour cream.

Day 25 menu

Breakfast
+ ¾ c. flake cereal C
+ 1 c. skim milk PD
+ 1 banana, sliced F
+ Calorie-free beverage

Lunch
+ **Tuna salad pita** V C PD Ft
  (Mix two 6-oz. cans of tuna packed in water, ½ c. diced celery, 2 tsp. lemon juice and ¼ c. low-fat mayonnaise. Place ¼ of recipe in ½ whole-wheat pita. Top with lettuce leaf, cucumber slices, and a tomato slice.)
+ 1 c. grapes F
+ Calorie-free beverage

Dinner
+ **Chicken Parmesan** C PD
  See recipe on this page. ✔
+ ½ c. cooked whole-grain pasta and ⅓ c. marinara sauce V C
+ ½ grilled zucchini drizzled with 1 tsp. olive oil V Ft
+ 1½ c. cubed watermelon F
+ Calorie-free beverage

Snack
+ 1 c. vegetable of choice V
+ 3 tbsp. fat-free ranch dressing Ft

Remember you can eat unlimited servings of vegetables and fruits.

Chicken Parmesan
+ Serves 4

4 (3-oz.) chicken breasts
2 egg whites
1 c. panko breadcrumbs
½ c. grated Parmesan cheese
2 tsp. dry basil
2 tsp. dry oregano
1 tsp. garlic powder
1 tsp. onion powder
2 c. marinara
¼ c. part-skim mozzarella cheese

1. Heat the oven to 375 F.
2. Pound chicken breasts to ¼-inch thickness and set aside.
3. Put egg whites in a small bowl.
4. Place panko breadcrumbs, Parmesan cheese, basil, oregano, garlic powder and onion powder in food processor. Process and pour mixture in another bowl.
5. Coat a baking sheet with cooking spray. Dip each chicken breast in the egg whites, dredge in the breading mixture and place on sheet. Bake about 15 to 20 minutes until golden brown.
6. Top with marinara and mozzarella cheese. Place back in oven until the cheese melts.

Week 4

Day 26 menu

Breakfast
+ **1 pumpkin spice muffin** `C` `PD` `S`
  See recipe on this page. ✔
+ **½ c. diced pineapple** `F`
+ **Calorie-free beverage**

Lunch
+ **Chicken Parmesan leftovers** `C` `PD`
+ **4 medium stalks celery** `V`
+ **¾ c. mandarin oranges** `F`
+ **Calorie-free beverage**

Dinner
+ **Macadamia nut crusted walleye**
  `F` `PD` `Ft` `Ft` `Ft`
  See recipe on page 298. ✔
+ **⅔ c. green beans** `V`
+ **1 small baked potato topped with
  1 c. steamed broccoli and
  ¼ c. salsa** `V` `V` `C`
+ **Calorie-free beverage**

Snack
+ **1 c. diced honeydew melon** `F`
+ **4 wheat crackers** `C`

Pumpkin Spice Muffins
+ Serves 14

2 c. pumpkin purée

2 c. plain fat-free Greek yogurt

2 eggs

¼ c. vegetable oil

1 tsp. vanilla

2½ c. flour

1½ c. sugar

1½ tsp. cinnamon

1 tsp. baking soda

1 tsp. ground cloves

¼ tsp. salt

1. Heat oven to 350 F.
2. Coat two muffin tins with cooking spray.
3. In a mixing bowl combine pumpkin purée, yogurt, eggs, vegetable oil and vanilla.
4. In another bowl combine flour, sugar, cinnamon, baking soda, ground cloves and salt.
5. Using a mixer, slowly combine the wet and dry ingredients until mixed well.
6. Scoop ¼ c. batter into each muffin well. Bake for approximately 25 to 30 minutes.

Week 4

Day 27 menu

V Vegetables	**PD** Protein/Dairy
F Fruits	**Ft** Fats
C Carbohydrates	**S** Sweets

Breakfast
+ ½ c. cooked oatmeal topped with
  1 c. milk and
  2 tbsp. raisins `C` `PD` `F`
+ ¼ c. mango `F`
+ Calorie-free beverage

Lunch
+ Quinoa cakes `C` `P` `Ft`
  See recipe on page 295. ✔
+ Salad `V` `V` `F` `Ft`
  (2 c. salad mix, 8 grape tomatoes, ¼ c.
  diced pepper, ½ c. sliced strawberries,
  4 tbsp. fat-free Italian dressing)
+ Calorie-free beverage

Dinner
+ 1 pita pizza `V` `C` `C` `PD` `Ft`
  See recipe on this page. ✔
+ ¾ c. mixed fruit `F`
+ Calorie-free beverage

Snack
+ 1 c. sliced bell peppers `V`
+ 2 tbsp. hummus `P`

Remember you can eat unlimited
servings of vegetables and fruits.

Pita Pizza
+ Serves 2

1 whole-wheat pita, cut in half
½ c. marinara sauce
½ c. diced red onion
¼ c. sliced mushrooms
¼ c. diced pineapple
¼ c. diced bell pepper
4 tbsp. part-skim mozzarella cheese
¼ c. reduced-fat feta cheese
2 slices chopped turkey bacon

1. Heat the oven to 375 F.
2. Coat a baking sheet with cooking spray and place the pitas on the sheet.
3. Divide ½ c. marinara sauce into the two pitas, and then divide the remaining ingredients between the two.
4. Bake 15 to 20 minutes or until the cheese is golden brown.

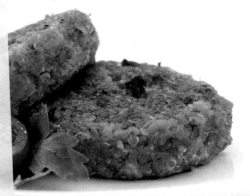

Week 4

Day 28 menu

Breakfast

+ 1 scrambled egg with ¼ c. salsa **V** **PD**
+ 2 slices whole-grain toast **C** **C**
+ 2 tsp. margarine **Ft**
+ 1 orange **F**
+ Calorie-free beverage

Lunch

+ **Roast beef wrap** **V** **C** **PD** **Ft**
  (2 oz. roast beef on a 6-inch tortilla with 1 c. sliced peppers, cucumbers and red onions and 2 tbsp. Italian dressing)
+ 15 cherries **F**
+ Calorie-free beverage

Dinner

+ **3 oz. salmon fillet, grilled** **PD** **Ft**
+ **1 c. roasted vegetable pilaf** **V** **V** **C**
  (Cook 1 c. brown rice with 2¼ c. water. Chop 2 c. each of onion, carrots and asparagus. Chop 1½ c. celery, and mince 2 tbsp. thyme. In a large nonstick skillet add 1½ tsp. olive oil and sauté the onion, carrot and celery until tender. Add the cooked rice, asparagus, thyme and 1 tsp. salt. Mix and serve.)
+ Calorie-free beverage

Snack

+ **Green smoothie** **F**
  See recipe on page 286. ✔

Dietitian's Tips

You can enhance the flavor of food without adding fat, salt or sugar. Herbs and spices contribute color, savory taste and sensational aroma:

+ **Basil.** An herb with a sweet, clove-like taste. Best used with Italian foods, especially tomatoes.
+ **Bay leaf.** A pungent, woodsy herb with a slight cinnamon taste. Best used with stews and soups.
+ **Caraway.** Seeds with a nutty, licorice flavor. Best used with beets, cabbage, carrots and turnips.
+ **Chili powder.** A commercial mix of chili peppers, cumin, oregano, and other herbs and spices best used with soups.
+ **Chives.** A member of the onion family with a mild onion flavor. Best used with baked potatoes, omelets, seafood and meat.

Week 4

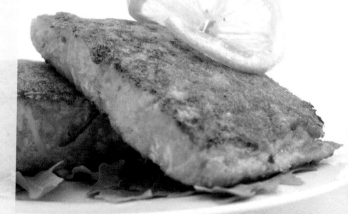

Index

A

ABC approach, 225–226

activity plan
 exercise buddy, 117
 expanding, 110–119
 fitness, 114–116
 keeping at it, 116–119
 obstacles, planning for,
  118–119
 overview, 111
 realism, 117
 time and schedule, 116–117
 See also physical activity

alcohol, 38, 171

all-or-nothing thinking, 232–233

apps, as tracking tools, 123

attitude, adjusting, 228–233

B

basal metabolic rate (BMR),
 156–158

behavior chains
 ABC approach, 225–226
 confrontation approach, 226
 defined, 223
 distraction approach, 226
 example, 223–224
 shaping approach, 228

behavior change
 celebrating, 231
 maintaining change, 207
 managing temptations and,
  209–210
 overview, 203
 planning ahead and, 208–209
 setting pace for, 207
 steps, 205–208
 stress and, 206, 210–211
 tips for, 208–211

behavior obstacles, action guide,
 248–255

beverages
 eating out, 196–197
 pyramid servings, 282–283
 in record keeping, 48–49

BMR (basal metabolic rate),
 156–158

body mass index (BMI)
 body fat and, 146
 defined, 144
 determining, 17, 145
 health risk and, 147
 in healthy weight, 144–146,
  148
 See also healthy weight

breakfast
 estimating servings, 104–105
 habit, starting, 23
 healthy, 22–23
 pyramid servings, 272–273

C

calories
 daily target, 85–86
 defined, 153
 empty, 157
 from fat, 151
 hidden, 194
 in *Live It!* phase, 85
 men average burn, 151
 pound of body fat equivalent,
  158
 in sample menus, 300
 servings and, 127
 sources of, 154–155
 tracking, 85, 152
 women average burn, 151

carbohydrates
 body use of, 154–155
 complex, 152–153
 gluten-free, 168
 highly refined, 264
 in Mayo Clinic Healthy Weight
  Pyramid, 166
 picking, 166

pyramid servings, 262–264
 simple, 152
 types of, 166

coffee, 196

confrontation approach, 226

D

daily goals, 56–57

daily servings, 86–87

dairy
 grocery shopping for, 175
 limiting, 28, 42
 low-fat, 43
 pyramid servings, 265–267
 See also protein

diabetes, 167

diets, special, 102–103

dinner
 estimating servings, 108–109
 ingredients, using for lunch,
  180
 pyramid servings, 276–278

distraction approach, 226

doctor, talking with, 17, 117

E

eating
 hunger and, 101, 210
 to pyramid and dining table,
  94–97
 slowly, 91
 stressed, depressed and
  bored, 251
 triggers, 232–233

eating out
 clues, uncovering, 191–194
 ethnic cuisine, 200–201
 extras, dealing with, 194–197
 at fast-food restaurants, 191,
  192–193, 199

PHOTO CREDITS

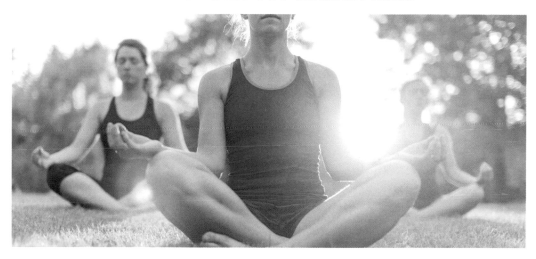

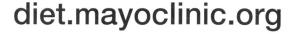

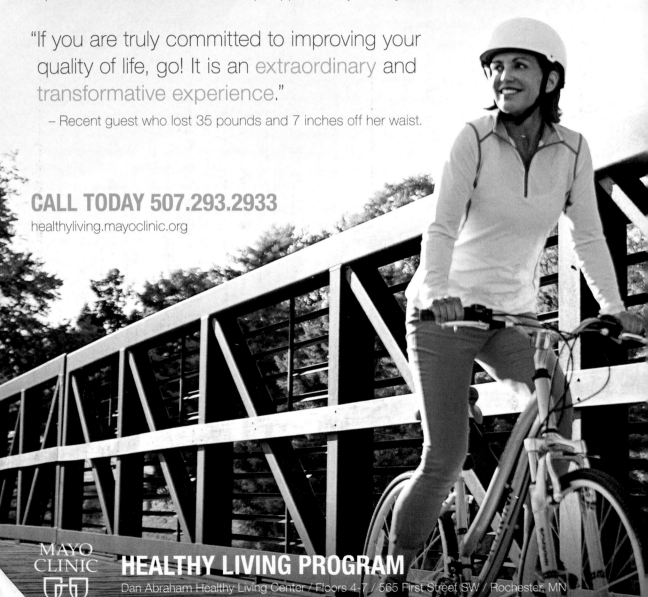

ACHIEVE YOUR WEIGHT-LOSS GOALS

The Mayo Clinic Diet Experience is an immersive weight-loss program that includes a 2-day on-site experience and 12 months of follow-up support from your Mayo Clinic certified wellness coach.

"If you are truly committed to improving your quality of life, go! It is an extraordinary and transformative experience."

– Recent guest who lost 35 pounds and 7 inches off her waist.

CALL TODAY 507.293.2933

healthyliving.mayoclinic.org

MAYO CLINIC

HEALTHY LIVING PROGRAM

Dan Abraham Healthy Living Center / Floors 4-7 / 565 First Street SW / Rochester, MN